The Hands Feel It

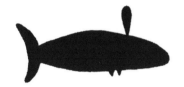

Healing and Spirit Presence

The Hands

among a Northern Alaskan People

Feel It

Edith Turner

NORTHERN ILLINOIS UNIVERSITY PRESS

DeKalb 1996

© 1996 by Northern Illinois University Press

Published by the Northern Illinois University
Press, DeKalb, Illinois   60115

Design by Julia Fauci

Turner, Edith L. B., 1921–
    The hands feel it : healing and spirit presence
among a northern Alaskan people /
Edith Turner.
        p.   cm.
    Includes bibliographical references and index.
    ISBN 0-87580-212-5 (cloth—alk. paper)
    ISBN 0-87580-573-6 (pbk.—alk. paper)
    1. Eskimos—Alaska—Medicine. 2. Eski-
mos—Alaska—Religion. 3. Ethnology—Field
work. 4. Spiritual biography. I. Title.
E99.E7T826 1996
299'.781—dc20   95-26638 CIP

Fran Durner photograph on cover courtesy of
Anchorage Daily News.

For Claire, Clem, and Netta

This book is their work

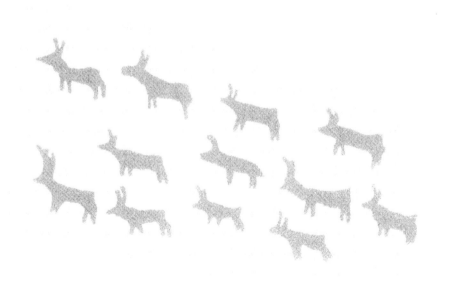

Contents

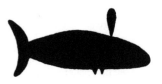

Acknowledgments

My warm thanks are due to my sponsors, the Wenner-Gren Foundation for Anthropological Research and the University of Virginia, and to Mary and James McConnell for further help. I am particularly grateful to the individuals to whom I have given the names "Claire Sivuq," "Clem Jackson," "Annie Kasugaq," and "Jim Agnasagga," all of whom were guides and educators in different ways. Clem declined coauthorship, though he was the theoretician behind this book. Claire intends to write a book of her own. I thank "Netta Jackson" in her flowery mountains, where she has now finally arrived. The people of Ivakuk gave me unstinted encouragement, help, and affection, which I remember with gratitude. I also give heartfelt thanks to all who assisted in the research in various ways, especially James Nageak, Theodore Mala, Rosita Worl, Lori Krumm, Karlene Leeper, Ann Fienup-Riordan, Judy Birckhead, members of the North Slope Borough, and many others.

I have done my best to reproduce conversations, events, and facts accurately; I apologize for the inadvertent errors to which a nonvillager (such as I) is prone.

To protect individuals and places in the field, I have used pseudonyms throughout the book, names taken at random from the Iñupiat region. I still respect the real names.

Families and Persons
Mentioned in Text

JACKSONS

Netta	great-great-grandmother, leading traditionalist, dancer, healer, author of oral histories
Kehuq	her senile husband
Kehuq	shaman, deceased, Kehuq's paternal grandfather
Clem	Netta's son's son, leading traditionalist, whaling captain
Margie	Clem's wife
Marco	Clem's son, clairvoyant
Lena	paternal cousin of Clem, expert in seal cutting
Kaglik	Netta's brother
Silas	Kaglik's son
Judy	Netta's mother's sister, a shaman, deceased
Runiq	Netta's mother's brother, a shaman, deceased

SIVUQS

Joanna	elder
Paula	her sister, deceased
Claire	healer, daughter-in-law of Joanna
Zeke	Claire's husband, whaling captain, adopted son of Joanna
Jeanie	adopted daughter of Claire and Zeke, learning healing

KASUGAQS

Annie	elder
Sam	Annie's husband, whaling captain, brother of Joanna Sivuq
Sam Junior	their son, deceased
Gordon	their son
Luanne	Gordon's girlfriend, mother of Gordon's children

LOWES

Seth	elder, whaling captain
Ezra	his brother, ailing, whaling captain
Dora	his sister, married to Robert Nashanik
Ardell	Seth's daughter, health aide
Elana	Ezra's daughter, store manager

NASHANIKS

Robert	son of Netta Jackson's sister, healer, whaling captain
Dora	Robert's wife
Catherine	daughter of Robert and Dora
Jimmy	son of Robert and Dora
Millie	Jimmie's girlfriend and mother of his child
Suellen	Robert's sister, healer
Ava	Suellen's daughter, healer

TUKUMAVIKS

Paula	deceased
Ed	son of Paula, language teacher
Edwina	Ed's daughter
Helen	Ed's sister, married to Tom Pingasut
Velma	Ed's sister

KUPERS

Agatha	an elder
Dick	her grandson, adopted as her son, boyfriend of the healer Ava, father of Ava's children

PINGASUTS

Tom	elder, whaling captain
Helen	his wife
Becky	their daughter
Ronnie	their son, deceased

AGNASAGGAS

Jim	biologist, nephew of Dora Lowe Nashanik
Naluq	his wife

OTHERS

Dionne Westfield	an elder whose home was built over shamans' graves
Peter	her grandson, adopted as her son

Aklak	an elder
Micky Hoffman	great-nephew of Aklak and grandson of a shaman; corporation legal adviser and later president of the Native Village of Ivakuk
Louis	Aklak's grandson
Michael	retired Iñupiaq preacher
Gabe	a whaling captain
Janet	a woman whaling captain
Don	her son, harpooner
Daniel North	postmaster
Jeanne	a teacher's aide
Mina	an elder
Madeline	an elder, "clown" of the village
Rafe Campesino	Chicano worker
Bruce Clay	White assistant to the borough mayor
Edie Turner	White anthropologist, elder
Carrie	White student
Marlene	White archeologist

Others are mentioned by name but appear only minimally in the account. For an alphabetical list of names, please see the index.

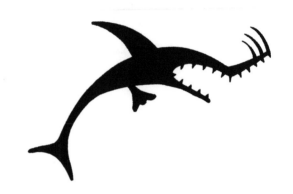

Introduction

In the far north of Alaska live a people related to the Inuit called the Iñupiat,[1] also known as Eskimos. These are a tough, hardy people, immensely practical, yet with a sense of spirits in the world. Although I had planned to study healing in one of their villages, soon after my arrival I saw that I would have to broaden the project and study spirit events as well. I spent a year there, from August 31, 1987, to August 15, 1988, and still make short visits every year. I joined in village life and wrote a journal that was both anthropological and personal. The present volume constitutes my Iñupiat chronicle.

As the fieldwork progressed, I became aware that my aim was veering toward the understanding of Iñupiat spirituality. The Iñupiat sometimes used this term as their most important characteristic: it referred to their experiences of spirit perception and the effectiveness of their spirit action generally, and it included Christian fundamentalist experience. The occasions of spirit events were indeed their high spots.

My method was to experience events as far as possible as the Iñupiat experienced them and to see the view from the inside in order to write those experiences; I saw the rootedness, the embeddedness of healing in their cosmos, a cosmos that included spirits. For them everything had a spirit, *iñua*, including not only what we call living beings, but also geographical features and even objects used in the general processes of life. While I was there I repeatedly heard from the villagers about spirit events, messages, and healings that they had experienced. Odd things happened to them and kept happening, and they sometimes happened to me, too.

The scene is a village I call Ivakuk,[2] a long way north of the Arctic Circle on the North Slope of Alaska—a wild country. The North Slope is so called because it is the slope that descends from the extreme northern end of the Rocky Mountain range northward to the long rim of the Arctic Ocean, taking in a broad region stretching from the Bering Straits to Canada.[3] The people of Ivakuk obtain two-thirds of their food from subsistence hunting, an activity they pursue on ice, sea, and land. In January 1988 the temperature went down to -30° Fahrenheit with strong winds. It was known as a warm winter. In summer it went up to about 55° Fahrenheit.

There are no trees at Ivakuk. Twenty miles toward the south small bushes appear in the river valleys, while a hundred miles south pines grow in sheltered places. That summer at Ivakuk I saw tiny purple, pink, white, and yellow flowers appearing between the pebbles, and later I saw some sea grasses. When I first arrived, I was struck by the flatness of the landscape. At Ivakuk, by the sea, the land is all gravel. The gravel bank on which the village stands extends for many miles to the southeast and ends in sea cliffs to the south. To the west it ends in a point far out in the ocean, from which the shore then sweeps back and continues in the same gravel bank to the northern cape far up the coast; it proceeds eastward from there along the North Slope in irregular fashion toward Canada. When I came to know the country, I realized how appropriate was the location of Ivakuk for the people's livelihood, because the whales and other sea mammals had no choice but to swim past the village on their annual migration east.

Well to the south there are fish camps for sporting Whites, heavily visited in the summer (sometimes the sportsmen fished in rivers that had been feeding Iñupiat—which provoked protests). Regular tourists would visit a neighboring center I name Bristol, to experience the midnight sun and view the museum. In the museum they could see beautifully laid out dioramas featuring snow and old-style kayaks, in which traditionally dressed Eskimo figures stood holding ivory weapons. The figures were surrounded by motionless animals of all kinds, including the white bear and the arctic wolf—nature, which so appeals to us. A live Eskimo dance troupe would perform for the tourists, demonstrating dances and the blanket toss, which latter is a feature of the traditional Whaling Festival. Tourists would admire the displays and envision the sea ice and the aboriginal world of the hunter.

Meanwhile, far to the north the village of Ivakuk was just itself, with no tourists, possessing its own non-Western history and numbering nearly seven hundred people, including a handful of Whites, settled in frame houses on the edge of the Arctic Ocean. Here the middle and senior elders still spoke their own language, though everyone also spoke English. They had their politics and their difficulties with the outside world and with each other, as people have elsewhere. Local politics was rich in its own right, in a style peculiar to Ivakuk Village. A major feature of local politics struck the Iñupiat whenever they walked out of the village: all along the coast could be seen the ruins of houses of precontact native peoples, 700 ruins, inhabited in the past by an average of 6 people in each, or a total of about 4,200 people. "There used to be 5,000 people here," said Clem Jackson, the most traditional of the Iñupiat traditionalists; 3,000, said Jim Agnasagga, the Iñupiaq biologist. By 1920 the population was reduced to 179, but since 1920 it has crept up again to 680. Large families are the rule.

The place and the ecology had its own ancient history concretized and present within it. A long time ago, when there was no land and no world, Tulungugraq, Raven, was paddling in his kayak on the sea. Tulungugraq noticed something dark under the water, rising toward him. He took his harpoon and struck. Then he pulled and pulled. The thing was very heavy. At last it showed, dark and big. A whale? It was the land, it was Ivakuk itself—it was the land and it was the whale too.

Many millennia passed while the people lived in their thousands along the shore and the river, in warm underground homes, with no government but the guidance of the elders. The hunting of sea mammals occupied their life; for this they used boats made of a driftwood frame covered with sealskin. These were passed down from father to son. Their tools and weapons were made of ivory and hard slate. On land they hunted caribou; the land was the territory of all. Here and there, however, out in the wilds, were spots that made people tremble to mention them, for a spirit was present there. The accounts of these were few but were matters of great seriousness. And so the people lived, using the products of the environment to feed a relatively stable population. They have been called peaceful, but over the centuries they have occasionally engaged in warfare.

Their shamans were both men and women. When the shamans used their abilities, the spirits and ancestors worked through them and performed the work of healing, changing the weather, finding lost people and objects, and communicating with the dead. These sessions took place in the neighborhood underground meeting house, *qalgi*. If a shaman wished to make a journey to cure a sick person, drummers and singers would assemble and sing the songs the shaman had taught them, who in turn had been taught them by his or her helping spirit. The shaman, in dancing his or her spirit animal, would eventually fall, and the shaman's spirit would depart, leaving the body behind. He or she would take a trip under the water or ice, or underground, or above the tundra, and would visit the home of the animals. There he or she would ask them to restore the sick person's health. In some cases a shaman might extract small spirit spear points from the patient's body by means of sucking where he or she perceived the trouble to be.

After centuries a new phase began in Iñupiat history. In 1850 White people arrived in Alaska with their commercial whaling ships, and by the next century most of the whales and other animals had disappeared. The people began to starve. Whites brought addictive substances to the village, substances that the civilized visitors thought were good: alcohol, tobacco, sugars, and refined flour products. These were made available in exchange for pelts. In addition to starvation and the ravages caused by addictive substances, the population was further reduced by all manner of diseases.

Among the newcomers was one who seemed to echo their own spirituality. In 1890 a strange White preacher turned up, who told them that God, clearly their Tulungugraq, had a son who had given himself for human beings. The White man preached for a time. Then, to the alarm of his missionary society, he took to drink, became an Iñupiaq, married, and went to live at the northern cape. The missionary society said he had become peculiar and replaced him, and we learn no more about him.

In 1939 and 1940 an archeologist and his colleague visited to excavate the old underground homes and graves in the area. He paid the Iñupiat villagers to work. His field notes contain detailed descriptions of human life at the time and tell how the missionaries were churlish toward poor young Netta Frankson, and how the Whites all sat on chairs in the public hall while the Iñupiat had to sit on the floor. The archeologist was indignant. Netta, although I came to know her well, never told me this story.

In the first half of this century severe epidemics struck the village, including influenza and measles, which were killers then, and tuberculosis, the most terrifying of the diseases. During the sixties and seventies the results of the oil boom overtook the people, and everyone was suddenly wealthy and very miserable. This time it was the culture that sickened. At the same time, because of sea erosion, the authorities moved the village to a new location, to an area with old funerary sites on it, but no one protested—then. To construct the new village, bulldozers first pushed thick gravel over the tundra, on the sites of the graves and on the summer grass, the flowers, and the pathways, in order to prevent mud conditions. The village was then built up on the gravel in a grid system of tarmacked streets, with a large school in the center.

During the later decades of the century the number of teenage suicides grew, reaching eight times the overall U.S. level, largely as a result of the school's penchant for training for jobs that only one-third of the students could obtain. This practice left them with an aim impossible to fulfill and thereby led them to substance abuse. Finally, from 1964 onward an epidemic of cancer began, which is now traceable to an experimental radioactive dump that was placed thirty miles from the village, without containers, on the best caribou feeding grounds. None of the Iñupiat knew about the dump until 1992, whereupon, after the Iñupiat had put much pressure on the government,[4] it was removed in 1993.

How did I find my way into this piece of local history? In 1986, shortly after I had been spending time in the midst of healing rituals in Zambia, two colleagues at the department of anthropology at the University of Virginia described a visit of theirs to the village I have called Bristol, where a huge gathering of all the Iñupiat had collected at the funeral of their leading healer. They reported that the healer had had many pupils.[5] As an anthropologist interested in ritual healing, I was intrigued. In 1987 I was able to take a leave from my university to go and study the healers myself. I arrived first in Anchorage and there met a student I will call Carrie, who was interested in being my future housemate. We flew north to Bristol and then by bush plane to Ivakuk. In the village itself we were assigned a tiny frame house. This was possible because I had made inquiries among friends that finally resulted in a connection with a family called Tukumavik, about which I knew nothing. A member of this family happened to own a house to rent. After I had lived there for a time, by dint of smiling a great deal and trying to behave with the courtesy and sharing behavior of the Iñupiat, I was gradually accepted in the village as a familiar, harmless figure, gray haired, an elder of sixty-six, with quite a number of children and grandchildren of her own living in the warmer zones of the world. And I regularly went to church.

I undertook this fieldwork suffering from various misconceptions. First, my intention was to specialize in Iñupiat healing and compare it with African healing. One of my associates was of the opinion, though, that Native Americans would not willingly talk about healing, which was probably a secret matter, so she advised me to collect life stories until I knew the village very well. But I found that healing was not secret. Second, I discovered that if I wanted to understand healing fully, specialization in healing alone would not suffice because at Ivakuk healing was an inseparable part of a wider phenomenon within the village—spirit perception and action. I needed to spread my attention to this broader sphere. I began with a third misconception: an expert on northern peoples had warned me it would take a whole year before I would begin to hear gossip—such was the reserve of hunting folks, he said. But the people of Ivakuk were different from those he knew. These gossiped a good deal. But gossip is dangerous material, and I have avoided it in this book. The people also took pleasure in telling me the strange events that occurred to them, and I am free to write about these because the most important representative of the "Native Village," Jim Agnasagga (having said, "Don't use our names"), urged me to give the village its true value in the face of the Whites. "Tell them that what we say is true. We need that," he said, referring to the Iñupiat experience of healing and spirit work. Consequently, I have set out the events that show their spirit work, events that actually happened. These were a topic of discussion beloved of Jim Agnasagga and me. In the following chapters I give accounts of some of our conversations.

The spirit experiences of the people are impossible to convey without the running story of everyday life because the experiences were embedded in human event, rooted in it, and the sense of the experiences might wither if I pulled them out of that earth. I work in an anthropological tradition substantially in line with Victor Turner's anthropology of experience (Turner and Bruner 1986), an anthropology that has been developing from Bakhtin's book on dialogics (1981) and from his stance on behalf of the primacy of the people (1965). My commentaries are often expressed in medias res, where they apply, just as spirit experience is best related in the context of ongoing life. My material is handled in the spirit of the natural historian, and because of a vivid sense of "being there," I have combined this handling with a degree of personal ethnography and a style related to anthropological poetics (Brady 1991).

One further remark, a caveat on the form and content of this book: although it is broadly in the form of a chronicle, obviously not everything that happened in the year is written here. I have been selective, favoring my chosen subject matter, and especially favoring the passages of life that ran the most warmly, much as an artist may sense in the landscape some kind of soul that she wishes to portray. Thus, to another visitor from the lower forty-eight states seeing Ivakuk for the first time, the village might seem banal and unappealing. Yet at an inner level the living tissues of it ramify as vividly and strongly as the life of a whale's body beats beneath many feet of flesh and fat.

The question of genre also arises. Is this anthropology? Anthropologists have the knack of entering the veins and arteries of the group itself and acting in unison with the people. Sometimes anthropologists make themselves into guinea pigs and let themselves loose, sacrificing their academic ego for experience, as Margaret Trawick (1990), Karen McCarthy Brown (1991), James Wafer (1991), and Kirin Narayan (1989) have done. In order to produce a genuine book this way, one needs to show the organic internal quality of the fieldwork itself, and let the material emerge as whole cloth, just as an unborn baby is itself and has not been "manufactured" inside the mother. Dennis Tedlock performed such a coalescence in his *Days from a Dream Almanac* (1990). These matters cannot be forced. They are what they are.

The book, then, has decided to emerge in the form of a year's chronicle. This is because the year's subsistence cycle was of paramount importance to the Iñupiat themselves. Different work and different hunting were done at different seasons, and the passing of the seasons decided the nature of every activity in the year and also influenced every episode of note in the village. My journals contained nearly all the field material I collected during the year-long visit. Continual tape recording, or writing field notes in front of my Iñupiat friends—except for more formal sessions—would not have fit their style. My conversations with the Iñupiat people were all unofficial, all human and merely friendly. My journal, written on the side, was full of what struck me about the events of the day, and I often used it to attempt to understand why such and such an event struck me so forcibly. I would write many comments on anthropological theory and make new theoretical explorations as they became relevant in the day-to-day work. These appear in the text at the date they were written because they were part of the development of the enterprise—which was to be conscious of the healing process and spirits. The journal also mentions connections with events in my previous researches; and it contains whole passages that are prose poems and recapitulations of strings of past events that make sense together.

Out of this I adopt a style like a novelist's but differing because I point to the society as hero, and especially to the activities of those people who manifested the curious gift of spirit perception and spirit action. Between the novel and anthropology there also lies another enormous difference. I did not make up this story. My account is not fiction. And its aim is not entertainment, but discovery and understanding.

Anthropological Forebears

Certain books and articles had a part in the way this volume was put together: Victor Turner (1967, 1974, 1975, 1986), Jean-Guy Goulet (1994), Michael Jackson (1989), Johannes Fabian (1983), Lucien Lévy-Bruhl (1985 [1910]), Ann Fienup-Riordan (1983, 1990, 1994), and Richard Nelson (1983), to name the strongest. These writings certainly corroborate what I found. They were a support, and I felt through them an ambience favorable to the research.

I realized that I needed to keep theoretical issues open. First, my previous work with Victor Turner and the mass of his work still in my littered study seemed to say, "Go by experience. Think about what you experience. Develop your ability to experience in different ways." In Victor Turner's work on experience he maintained that experience was primary and that objectified mind, that is, laws and culture, were secondary (see Turner and Bruner 1986).

I began to develop my ability to experience in Africa in 1985, and I explain the process in E. Turner (1992). My experience of seeing a spirit, there related, forms the next basis from which I addressed this research, which is the nondenial of and a positive interest in the existence of spirits. In Zambia I saw the traditional doctors trying to pull an afflicting spirit out of the body of a sick woman. For that task they used cupping horns and worked their ritual to draw the spirit into a horn. At the climax of the drumming and singing, after many attempts, it suddenly became clear that the spirit was actually coming out. And at that point I saw with my own eyes a large gray ball, something between solid and smoke, a kind of globular ghost, emerge from her back. The doctors put whatever it was into a bag and later showed it; then it appeared to have taken the form of a tooth. They fed the tooth with blood and meal, and the woman recovered. Having seen this thing, I understood that Africans were likely to be right about spirits, and by extension, perhaps the Iñupiat were right about theirs.

I realized that I should be careful about using the word *myth* for their narratives. An Iñupiaq intellectual has asked me not to use the words *story, legend,* and *fable* about her people's history, words that might imply it was not true. I agreed to refrain. Of course I do not claim that the rest of the world has to abide by what the Iñupiat say. There then arises the problem of how differing histories can all be true. This book exists under the shadow of that problem. Within the network of Iñupiat life one becomes aware of the Iñupiat's own truth, *in process,* in use (see Jackson 1989). There is a particular role for ethnography, a role now practiced extensively, that draws close to the personal among people of different societies, whoever they are.

A matter I had been learning in conversation with the ordinary people of America formed a third aspect of my thinking. In a much later essay of Jean-Guy Goulet (1994) on the Dene Tha of northwest Alberta, Goulet describes how he made the discovery that if one tells one's own story and includes what is deepest to oneself, one will get back some very serious and true accounts of quite unusual matters that are of prime importance to the other teller. Goulet found that "what the Dene view challenges us to do is to produce stories much as they do, stories that express personal life experiences in the Dene world as they conceive of it and seek to live it" (Goulet 1994, 122). Coexperiencing, then, is of the essence in this kind of research, as Victor Turner said:

> My counsel, therefore, to investigators of ritual processes would be to learn them in the first place "on their pulses," in coactivity with their enactors, having beforehand shared for a considerable time much of the people's daily life and gotten to know them not only as players of social roles, but as unique individuals, each with a style and a soul of his or her own. Only by these means will the investigator become aware of the communitas in the social structure. (1975, 28–29)

In addition, it must be understood that none of this research material can live without its soil—that is, attention to context, social setting, the ongoing life of the people, even social dramas (those that are printable). The tensions, the contemporary anomalies, all are actually needed to get the sense of such a thing as a healing, and what the people are feeling. And for the interpretations of spirit events, I was ready to turn to the people's own interpretations after having come to understand how appropriate they were in the case of the Ndembu of Zambia.

Victor Turner used the terms *context sensitive* and *context general* about ritual, particularly religious ritual. A church service repeating old forms was context general, whereas a Zambian healing ritual especially for an individual was context sensitive. The events I examine are context sensitive. Parallel to this, Michael Jackson's work later showed how ritual is "true" in the context in which it is "used" (Jackson 1989). Now this is profound. The usual policy of using "the scientific method" in order to prove something is true is out of the picture here. Here we are down to warm bodies, full emotional human beings, and a strange thing called ritual action, which intervenes and alters the situation on the spot. The question is, how does it do it?

Johannes Fabian (1983) provides another theoretical basis, showing that anthropologists now have to consider the people they study to be in the same world and to be influenced by the same forces as the researchers, with the same consciousness of the times in which they live. The people we study are not frozen in a present tense; they are coeval with us. He taught that the attribute of co-evalness was the right of all humanity. We should not treat anthropological field people as specimens. For instance, a missionary in Zambia said, "The African likes his meat bad"—present tense. In other words, "he" is a generalized savage, does not live in the same world as us, and does not progress as we do. My Iñupiaq friend Jim Agnasagga and I live passionately in the same world. And we live in the same time, time that eats away the old and brings grandchildren to both of us. Jim has built up my field methods for me.

Another obvious forebear is old "Uncle Lucien" Lévy-Bruhl. He examined the masses of material on undeveloped peoples in strange lands who came under study at the turn of the twentieth century, whose thinking was "prelogical." Lévy-Bruhl showed that the people he studied lived by "the law of mystical participation" (1985)— a statement worthy of a Hasid. His work, like that of Arnold van Gennep, both marginal to the Année Sociologique school of French rationalism, has continued to develop through a number of anthropologists. What Emile Durkheim, the French school's leader, who derived all human action from humanity's social environment, has given us is deconstructionism, if that helps. Eighty-five years after Lévy-Bruhl I find my friend Claire, an Iñupiaq healer, living by the law of mystical participation. It does not go away. In her world there is often a network of this participation. Desjarlais says of Nepalese healing that the healing takes place within an ecology of knowledge, a collective circuit of knowledge. The flow that includes the Yolmo patient, the shaman, and the gods forms part of, and works toward, that ecology. "The larger ecology 'knows' about such matters at some tacit level," says Desjarlais (1992, 184).I realized that the whole of things has this reticular nature, just as the theory of relativity teaches, because the network, the whole array, moves. In Alaska Ann Fienup-Riordan (1983, 1990, 1994) has expounded the milieu in which the Yup'iit people (southern Eskimos) live—a cosmos within which animals cycle into the bodies of humans, the humans reincarnate and replenish the cosmos, and all objects of the cosmos are living souls, some of them cycling more slowly, but in their proper courses. Fienup-Riordan's book (1994) confirmed for me what I was finding further north.

Furthermore, unknown to me, an old rationalist, Richard Nelson (1983) had been turning around and seeing the Koyukon Indian hunters of Alaska as equal to and not above the animals, and extraordinarily in touch with them. Nelson, no longer a rationalist, found himself at last making prayers to Raven, as I was learning to do. This "conversion" of his strengthened my writing.

Finally, I should mention those in anthropology who have themselves written, sometimes extensively, about the spirit experiences they have shared with people in the field. Their work is growing in volume. I include Stoller (1989, 37–56), who experienced witchcraft in Niger; Favret-Saada (1980), who also experienced witchcraft in rural France; Grindal (1983), who saw a dead man rise up and dance in Ghana; Peters (1981) and Desjarlais (1992) who went into shamanic trance themselves in Nepal; Evans-Pritchard (1937, 11), who saw a spirit light among the Azande; Bowen (1954), who saw witchcraft in Nigeria; Laderman (1991), who experienced the spirit wind of the Malays herself; Goulet (1994), who had prophetic dreams in the field in South America, and saw visions among Northern Canadian natives; Marton (1994, 277–79), who saw a spirit light in the context of the study of Afro-Cuban Santeria; Young (1994), who saw visions of spirit visitors after participating in Cree sweat lodges; McCall (1993), who had a prophetic dream in Nigeria; and Salamone (1995), who experienced the clairvoyance of a medicine man in Nigeria. In the anthropology of religion one may mention Guédon (1994), who had prophetic dreams among the Dene of Alaska, Hultkrantz (1992, 91), who was healed by a Shoshone medicine man, and Brown (1991), who participated in Voudou. There are plenty of others, many of whom have not published their material.

In all, I see much support for experiential anthropology and many advances in it. The authors to whom I have referred in this introduction were the antecedents of the present study, and their work applies more specifically to the particular nature of this research than any other. Anthropology has been much influenced by the French structuralists and also by Kant, before Lévi-Strauss, who argue that culture is derived from systems of archetypes in the human mind—in Kant's case called "noumena" and in Lévi-Strauss's, "structures." Curiously, I can now see these very archetypes as spirits and am interested in what these thinkers were groping toward. But Lévi-Strauss's work sometimes became disturbingly intellectual and over-logical, contradicting his own brilliant insights. To counteract the old ideas about archetypes, some anthropologists, the deconstructionists, have tried to tear off the structures and return to the idea of the "empty slate" beginning of all humanity, filled throughout by "social constructions of reality." But there are people inside those societies that have wondering and vulnerable souls, people who are *in* the society yet not in it—actually thinking. Fortunately, I did not go by way of the structuralist, constructionist, or deconstructionist theoretical schools. I approached my study through process anthropology, and I was glad, moreover, that Clifford (1983) and his school advocated that anthropologists should put themselves into the picture.

Summary of Propositions Derived from the Iñupiat Research

My attention first focused on the way to bear the living gift of Ivakuk out to the world. For me, a fruitful method arose from the wellsprings of the Iñupiat themselves, not by means of interviews, or the amassing of facts in categories, or studying ancient accounts. For instance, it is possible to relate some of the features of the present-day links between humans, animals, and spirits to records of earlier Iñupiat ethnography.[6] But rather than comparing these accounts point by point, I reveal the present-day culture in action. For every era is different, and every era takes from the previous one what is alive. There have been numerous accounts of animals communicating with people in the history of Ivakuk, many of them influencing the present culture; the power of this culture in the last analysis, though, is in the Now. Therefore, one needs to be alert for continual changes and unexpected subtleties in that Now. The anthropologist Michael Jackson would call this method "epistemic pluralism," which

> suggests an opportunistic, improvisatory attitude to ethnographic enquiry. Truth is seen pragmatically, not as an essence but as an aspect of existence, not as some abstraction such as Science, Rationality, Beauty, or God, to be respected whatever the circumstances, but as a means of coping with life. . . . Can our discourse be likened to . . . a game we play with words, the thread of an argument whose connection with reality is always oblique and tenuous, which crosses to and fro, interlacing description with interpretation, instruction with entertainment, but always ambiguously placed between practical and antinomian ends? If so, truth . . . is in the interstices as much as it is in the structure. (1989, 185–86, 187)

What appears in this book is a contemporary operative play of events. I cannot call the elements I have selected for attention "a set of concepts," or even "symbols" with such and such "meanings." What I show is a moving, working process. My first proposition, therefore, is action, action itself, discovered by *working* under the aegis of the Iñupiat, embedded in village life—and afterward the writing of Iñupiat action as a record parallel to the living scene.[7]

As a corollary proposition to the policy of searching for the context-sensitive in this manner, a point needs to be made about the problem involved in creating overly sharp definitions, particularly of soul, spirit, breath, the entity that reincarnates, the spirit in the body that responds to the healer's hands, and so on. Even to define these at all would seem to involve generalizations that would overload spirit activity with cognitive thinking. Spirit activity works in the immediate situation and is understood in its living context. Definitions and theologies tend to prevent the likelihood of spirit healing because they intellectualize entities that are not mental but are of spirit stuff.

And from this comes proposition three (only a proposition, not a law), that one needs to develop a sense of how one's spirit milieu may change, a sense of discrimination among the different levels, the ability to prick up one's ears. A society can flow easily from one level to another as the fluctuations within a level may run over into another. This is much more common than we suppose and takes place often in my account.

I saw too how chance, the random play of events, the fluid stance of a hunter, the flashes of odd circumstances coming together, were what regular life was made up of in Ivakuk and how they provided a poetic and extraordinarily open character to almost everything that happened. (Oddly enough, this came out strongly in bingo.) In a hunting and gathering village that has had the bureaucracy of the state imposed upon it, there occurs the whirling against each other of two systems—similar to the typical circumstances covered by chaos theory. I have called it the churning effect. Chance, divination, the unexpected, and the hunter's life were typical and likely circumstances that would promote spirit entry.

Finally, as the year went on, the threads of connectedness became more obvious—in the kinship and pseudokinship system, in healing, in the form of the language, in the relation of old to young, and in the small histories always being passed down to the young. These connecting threads were obvious—literally—in the making of clothes and the connecting of seams (immensely important), as well as in subsistence hunting itself—namely, the connection between human and animal. The vagaries of chaos, the churning effect, spun their own mysterious "strange attractor," an ever tighter cocoon of connection.[8] Many were the spirit matters that involved connectedness or needed it to flourish: cosmological cycling, spirit communication, animal spirits, the transformation of an evil spirit animal into a good one, reincarnation, the meaning of the multifaced carved mask, the shaman's four-day fugue syndrome, the "conversation of bodies" in healing, near-death experiences, the awareness of ghosts, the transcending of clock time, chance, prophetic dreams, and even the tradition that the world was once upside down compared to what it is now. When connected, animals teach humans, not the other way around. Spirits exist, in particular the self-sacrificing spirits of the whale and eagle, and they extend themselves through humans into the cycling process, which has to continue.

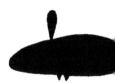

The Hands Feel It

1
Arrival

August 31, 1987, Monday. Carrie (my student friend) and I were flying north along the seacoast from Bristol to Ivakuk. I couldn't believe the landscape below on my right—it was unearthly, as if we were flying over another planet. It seemed to consist of gray rolling tides of barren ground, as if the earth had been razed by immense forces and then just left. Drifts of snow lay here and there even though it was late in the summer. After nearly an hour spent steadily rounding the coast, we passed a range of sea cliffs, beautiful in their stark declivity, then flew beside a long, long coastline backed with a maze of curving lagoons, graceful to see. It was a geometric world, a land with no sign of life. I was seeing the hand of nature. Now the coast curled westward out into the sea, and I saw that we were flying toward a distant extended point of land where two converging coasts met and became nothing, a nothing that curled a little more still and gave way immediately to another northern sea. Where were we going? We crossed over into the northern space, and then our small plane turned staggeringly and shot downward in the direction from which we had come. Almost at once we were riding on land, with tarmac and yellowed grasses on either side. At the end of the airstrip we slowed. A shed came into view, also a bus and a truck, and here the plane came to a halt. The White pilot climbed out and released the steps. He brought out our luggage, which consisted of suitcases, a sleeping bag, and stuff bags containing clothes, bulk oatmeal, bulk rice, and bruised bananas. A middle-aged brown man in a warm jacket and pants pointed to the parka I was carrying on my arm. "You put on your jacket."

I thought, "Yes"—for a chilly wind was blowing. I put it on gratefully. I was excited but tried not to show it. The man directed Carrie and me to the bus, and we clambered up into it with our luggage, accompanied by the Iñupiat people who had been our traveling companions on the plane. They included a couple on their way back from the hospital with a recovering baby. As we had been instructed, we asked the Iñupiaq driver to go to "Tom Pingasut's house."

"You an elder?" he said to me.

"Yes. I'm sixty-six," I said.

"An elder. You don't have to pay." My friend Carrie was twenty-two and paid fifty cents. We bumped along to the village, all of us chatting. The speech around me was in English, in the falling tones of Native Americans, bursting into laughter at intervals. I began to chat too, eagerly, in my elder's way, and felt cheerful. Whatever kind of fieldwork this was going to be, at least it was pleasantly sociable. Out of the corner of my eye I could see the reality of the map I had been studying. The long shingle, just as the map had shown, stretched as far as eye could see. Then the road seemed to pass through an army dump of gray objects set on the gravel, with huge oil tanks off to the left. Okay. There was a bit of grass. This was a human environment just as Chicago was a human environment. I had liked Chicago. I was determined to find this exciting.

We reached a prosaic clutch of small prefabs, each with a dump around it. This was Ivakuk. Almost at once we were at Tom Pingasut's door. We knocked. His wife Helen was in; she was a small Iñupiaq in modern clothes, that is, a blouse and pants. She was the person to whom I was supposed to apply for the key of the house we were renting.

Helen had a gentle, wrinkled face with Asiatic eyes. She told me, "We'll have to wait for Becky. She has the key. I forgot you were coming today." We had phoned Helen Pingasut, saying we needed a place in Ivakuk so that we could talk to the elders. I had not yet mentioned healing. Maybe the Iñupiat would not communicate about such a thing unless one were a very special person, which I certainly was not. I would have to learn the sense of the community as regards healing.

We waited in Helen's living room for a while, not saying much to her. We were sitting on a couch; there was a TV, and family group photographs adorned the walls.

Helen volunteered, "Agatha Kuper's in charge of the Senior Citizens Center here—they have a lunch once a week on Saturdays."

"Thank you." Privately I thought, "So the senior citizens have been organized into a group. Okay."

Becky arrived and turned out to be an active young woman in a sports jacket and pants. Apparently no one wore dresses here. Becky took us by bus with our luggage to the rented house, a little frame dwelling raised off the gravel on posts. A rusty oil tank was suspended near the door. We struggled with the key in the locked door, but it was the wrong key. Becky marched around the house to a back window. She tried the window; then with a strong arm she wrenched the whole frame away and called her little son to climb in and open the front door.

I looked at the wrenched window. Carrie said, "Thank goodness I brought the duct tape. We can seal the window back in again." (Carrie's experience with Northwest Coast Indians had taught her to be practical. She was engaged to marry an Indian, a handsome dark-haired young man named Buddy.) Carrie was a woman of much presence and beauty. Her hair was long and golden brown. I myself, clumsy, active, gray-haired, didn't know what presence I had and didn't care much.

Becky lit the oil stove with waste paper and then left. We peered around at the spotted carpet and the dirty dishes piled in the sink. They could wait. Meanwhile I sighed, feeling the relief I always felt when I was at home. We unpacked our stores and made a meal, then found our way on foot to the Ivakuk Native Corporation store. At last we had a chance to go out and see where we were. Up until now we had been rushed from point to point, seeing areas of gray gravel, various workaday prefab houses, nothing except the utilitarian. It was no different as we walked, making our way down a grid system street under a gray sky, with wide gravel stretches on each side and prefab houses placed at intervals. The road needed repair. We were shy of the people who passed by dressed in their warm jackets. I noticed the tang of sea air in the place.

The store was in the middle of the village, past the fifty-foot water holders, the power station all athrum, the little prefab clinic, and the laundromat. The store beyond stretched out in long, prefab style, set on gravel like everything else. It was painted blue. Carrie and I crunched toward the wooden steps of the store, climbed up, and passed through a long passage. Inside, we strolled around the aisles, finding the shelves almost bare save for some packets of fancy noodles, some bags of sugar, and some photograph albums. [The native store was owned by the Ivakuk Native Corporation, and the corporation was in Chapter 11, near bankruptcy, for reasons that became clear to us later.] And I saw something I didn't quite understand: in spite of this trouble that affected the whole village, the people we encountered were buoyant and cheery.

We returned to the counter. I began telling the Iñupiaq store clerk that I was there to hear the elders' stories. She pointed out a small person and said, "That's Netta Jackson." We drew near. "She teaches Iñupiat dancing in the school. She tells stories."

A tiny, active woman in her late seventies, wearing a colorful parka, stood before us with her face upturned, murmuring disclaimers. I gathered from what she said that I might be able to see her dancing. She said nothing about stories, and I didn't press it.

At this point my mind was energized by our logistic problems. We would have to find the post office and send a mail order for food. I would have to find language instruction. I would need to install in our house a Citizens Band radio box with a mike and small antenna. Most of the villagers used these to speak to people in other houses, and whale hunters used them to send messages about the animals.

One is like a newborn baby in such circumstances, decanted into a strange world and probably having that vague look of a newborn baby who is innocently taking things in. Out of the window I could see small Iñupiat women toddling about on the loose gravel and could hear them call each other by their first names. Sometimes we could see people swinging by, mounted on all-terrain vehicles open to the sky, machines called Hondas. These vehicles consisted of three heavy balloon-type wheels, a motor bicycle engine, handlebars, a motor-bike seat, a rack behind, and that was all. Who the various people that passed were I did not know.

Thus we began our life in Ivakuk, sometimes talking to the store assistant and sometimes to Daniel, the postmaster.

September 5, Saturday. I had been looking forward to this Saturday because I could follow Helen Pingasut's advice and attend the elders' lunch, free of charge at the local "hotel," which consisted of a diner with a shack motel behind it, offering rather plain rooms, for which the motel charged visiting White construction workers $150 a night. I was the first of the elders to arrive at the diner. As I drank my coffee, the elders turned up in a special "senior van" bus. They stumped in cheerfully, then each one stripped off her non-zip-front parka by bending and bundling it over her head. They seemed an active bunch, none of them crippled or in pain, but they were small. The women had flat, wrinkled faces and beady eyes and were direct and practical in manner. The two men present looked pleasantly whimsical and even a little dangerous. One of the women was Joanna Sivuq, a person with squidgy eyes and a difficult way of speaking English. In order to be friendly I brought out some photographs from my purse and showed Joanna some pictures of my half-Chinese grandchildren Benjamin and Daniel. She said indifferently to her neighbor, "*Taniq*" (Whites). I had been hoping she might say they were like Iñupiat.

I sat eating. I began to think of what I had read concerning events in Ivakuk in the 1970s, when the whole village had been forced to move to a new site owing to sea erosion at its old site. I asked Joanna which was the better place, the old village they had left behind at the end of the beach, or the present one.

"*That* one," she said, meaning not this.

I asked Joanna if her daughter-in-law, Claire, the healer, was in town, or was she at fish camp?

"No. She'll be home for a while."

The meal was over. Joanna toddled off to look out for the senior van that was going to take them home. When it arrived they all piled in chattering in Iñupiat, everyone in a good mood. I followed them into the van. One old man was roaring with laughter from some carefully thought-out joke. As soon as the joke was circulated among the rest of the elders, the van was in pandemonium. I grinned feebly, but it meant nothing to me. Eventually the bus set me down at my door.

Certain families had indeed been at fish camp. Carrie and I looked out of our window and saw a Honda all-terrain three-wheeler arrive at the house opposite. A man and some boys climbed off it. One of the men carried a heavy, tall white bucket up the steps of the porch of the house, through the door, and into the inner porch. More small boys came out of the house and danced around. Very good cheer reigned. An older woman came out. The children went to a hut set back from the big house, and out of that hut came a younger woman with a baby on her back. She entered the main house. After some time the man came out of the main house swinging the bucket, which was now obviously empty. A small boy of about three remained outside casting something on a line—he was "fishing." Shortly afterward, to my surprise, the older woman came around to my house carrying a fish. She presented me with the fish, introduced herself as Annie, and complained that we hadn't visited her. We thanked her and shared a cup of tea. Annie was a fat, cheerful woman with short black curly hair. Her face kept looking up at me frankly; I looked back at her with my own frank face. I liked her but could scarcely understand what she was saying because of her strong accent.

September 6, Sunday.   Carrie had not been idle. I did not know it, but she had quickly made friends with three teenage girls. Little did I know what we were in for late that night. The three girls came to visit us to watch Carrie do beadwork. I had already gone to bed, but I heard them come because my room was nothing more than a cubicle in the small house, with a gap between the partition top and the ceiling.

Carrie was at work at the table. "Hi, Edwina." The girls gathered around.

They were discussing ear-piercing to take bead earrings, and the conversation went on to lip-piercing. When I heard the first sentence behind the partition I reached for my notebook and took down the words verbatim. The voice seemed to be mourning in tone, even poetic. I was getting used to this Native American tone; the girl was eager and intense, with a trace of teenage show-off.

". . . my great-great-grandmother put a tattoo on me when I was five years old," I heard in the gentle sing-song. "It was a heart. She did it by needling. I was the only one in the family she did it to. I cried 'cause it hurt. They were wondering why she did it. *She* was laughing, *I* was crying. She forced it on me. Every time I look at my tattoo it reminds me of my great-great-grandmother; she was kind of like a spirit doctor."

"Spirit doctor?" said Carrie.

"Shaman."

"Are they still around?"

"They're all dead. You can uncover them in the graves and see the bones. You're not to touch them. One of them used to try to rape her."

"The spirit doctor tried . . . ?" I could hear Carrie jump up.

"There's a man who had a spell put on him."

[Carrie explained this afterward: "A kind of spirit war was going on, some of this stuff you cannot analyze and name. It goes like this; it's simple: the woman and the man were both medicine doctors. He was trying spiritually to rape her, and she turned around and cast a spell on him, and he became crazy."]

Now Edwina's singsong, high-toned voice continued: "There's a haunted house in Traderstown [a beach up the coast where international commercial whalers used to land and trade whiskey, rum, sugar, flour, and ammunition, in exchange for pelts]. Someone almost got killed last week. He was drunk; he tried to go to sleep in one of these old houses and was almost choked to death. It really *freaks me out.* I don't like to sleep in those places." I shuddered, listening.

"You're supposed to say nothing about shamans, not even touch their graves, or they'll harm you. Me, her, and Kagak, and Rafe and Amy [these latter were the Chicano father and Iñupiaq mother of the girl named Kagak], we noticed a person walking on air, floating. We realized he wasn't walking like a normal person. 'C'mon Rafe, don't, stop it, don't do that,' I said, thinking it was Rafe scaring me. But no, the person was on the lake, and all of a sudden it was behind us. We started running!

"Rafe liked to take us down to the shaman graves; they like us to know our history, like. That person was floating in the air. Amy knows about it.

"There was that hooked man, half man, half woman, like the devil with caribou legs. Three months ago my dad saw it at night by our campsite. And he saw it in black walking down here by that house next door, the one where the man shot himself. The man shot himself because the hooked man made him crazy. Stella Jackson, a true Christian, she saw it, that black thing. It went right by her window and laughed at her. She prayed, you know, prayed, and it disappeared and passed over." The voice was lowered in awe. I goggled behind the wall.

Lori said, "Is it the Sasquatch?"

"Not it. There are little people, you know, nine- and ten-foot, fifteen-foot people, in Tuviq there. My dad saw green little people, tall little people. Amy *freaked out!* They went way out in the ocean. I was only eight or nine at the time. Those tall green people like to get young kids, I'm telling you. We were in a boat, so our mothers and fathers covered us with caribou skins as it was *scary.* They threw sleeping bags over us. We had to go five or six miles out to sea to get away from them. That was 'our history,' yecch! Green people and little people, ten-footers, medicine persons, left over from the tundra in 1300 or 1500. When they get a person they cut 'em up and eat 'em raw. Bit scary. God!" (in tones of awe).

I was scribbling fast, hooked on the wild narrative myself, and puzzled in particular about the anomaly, "little tall" people. Meanwhile, the girl's eyes evidently fell on some Iñupiat language flash cards that Carrie and I had left spread out on the table.

"You'll learn it," said Edwina tolerantly, then returned to her narrative.

"Ronnie Pingasut shot himself when he was sixteen years old because of a girl. [This event took place in the house next door to ours.] The girl was trying to mess with Ronnie's mind. He shot himself with a .22 gun. The bullet traveled inside his head. It happened in the back room over there, in 1978. Man, it was nine years ago. So fast! Nine years ago; it went by so fast."

I took a breath. Edwina certainly had a talent for storytelling. "Freaks me out," was her favorite phrase. [Reading my notes later, I wondered whether I had been presented with all my fieldwork on spirit perception during the first weekend. I was fascinated by the green tall little people, for a start. I had heard of the little people and giant people from Burch's article on the Iñupiat (1971). So these creatures apparently changed size as well as shape. Why not change size indeed? What is scale, after all?]

These high school students were accepting their "history," as they called it, and being repelled by it at the same time.

September 7, Monday.   Here was a prefabricated village deposited upon the gravel, yet I knew it had roots; it had a past out there. Those roots were in the cemetery, I knew—a place to which I could at least walk, visit the graves, and pay my respects—and this way I would be able to make some kind of connection, do something real. So this day Carrie and I tried it. We started out, plodding over the gravel and grass west of town. Almost immediately rain and snow began to fall, so that my feet soon got wet. I huddled into my light raincoat and thin scarf, but it was ultimately the wind rather than the cold that got to me. [It took me another month to learn sense and acquire a homemade contemporary Iñupiat parka, in high Ivakuk style, fashioned from printed velveteen with a padded lining, windproof, complete with a wolverine hood that really kept the wind out.] Still poorly protected, we shivered as we walked toward the cemetery, making our way first to a giant whale jawbone, erect and solitary on the land. In all the expanse there was nothing left of the summer save one tiny purple flower emerging from a four-inch pad of tiny leaves. When we arrived at the jawbone, we saw that it was actually set there as a monument, with a grave at its foot. The grave was glassed over and enclosed a large wooden cross dimly visible beneath. Under the glass we could see many wreaths of artificial flowers and a paper with illegible writing. Walking further, we found the cemetery itself, a wide area fenced in by whale ribs. We went around and entered by two tall jawbones. The place was filled with wooden crosses and giant upright bones. Most of the crosses bore no names, although a few had a name and a simple Bible verse. The blankness of the unnamed ones made me feel lost. Many crosses were adorned with bright pale-colored artificial flowers. On this day of rain, snow, and wind streaking across the moorland, as we stood within the shelter of the whale rib fence, the flowers made a strange contrast—they were unreal, gay, even emotionally moving. I did pay my respects: I prayed beside a randomly selected grave for the Ivakuk people.

We walked on. A mile beyond the cemetery appeared the airstrip, and immediately beyond that we began to see the dilapidated houses of the old town site: the school house, the mission site, the meeting hall, and among many other ruined homes the shaman's house, full of trash. Poking inside one particularly strange snow-filled house we discovered at the far end of the living room a derelict piano banked up with old snow. I gazed sorrowfully at the pitted polish on the piano lid and peered inside to where the banks of wires half emerged from settled snow. We found out later that this was Netta Jackson's old house and that the piano had been hers. We left the house and wandered further on still, toward where the sea seemed to draw near to us. We were seven miles from home and there was not much further we could go. Large mounds appeared here and there. We came across one that was concave in the middle and saw that the roof had caved in. Whale ribs protruded from it in a circle; they must have been the rafters. To the inhabitants it must have seemed like living inside the whale. In a sense it was. Another mound appeared with an entrance tunnel ending in a squat wooden door frame, on the side post of which a ceramic telephone wire holder had been screwed. The tunnel of this one was also caved in. The entrance to yet another was still intact, and we could go in. We could see how the roof of the tunnel was entirely lined with whale ribs and scapulas. We struggled through the tunnel and turned a corner into a storage space. It was warm in here. I could see that the corner helped to break the draft. Another tunnel appeared in front with turf showing between the whale bone rafters. At the far end a real room appeared, where the air was chilly because the skylight, the room's one window, was without its covering; it had neither the old style seal guts sewn together nor glass. We were in a square room, with boards for walls and flooring, a room constructed after the mission fashion. We found a tiny table in one corner on which lay a child's music book, and in another corner an elegant hoop-backed chair. We retreated to the first tunnel and observed tiny mouse-like footprints in the snowdrift just within the entrance. They were lemmings' footprints, looking busy and homey. Carrie, who was a meditator, sat for some minutes in the lotus position on this spot, but all I could do was hunker down and gaze affectionately at the footprints.

Emerging again among the mounds, we walked onward, now over curling shingle down to the end of the beach. Here for ages past the sea had been eating away the land of the north shore and giving it to the south shore. Carrie remarked that the hook at the end, curling toward the left, had created a kind of yin-yang sign between the water and the land. Because it was low tide, we found we could stand way down at the hub of the hook, deep within a wide cup of roiled sand, the hub being the water eye of the yin-yang sign. It felt deeper than it was, a self-made place. Was I intruding? Then we went and stood on the high central knob spun from the high tide at the other eye of the sign, the land eye. The whole point was in a continual state of eating and being eaten.

As for the Iñupiat people, they regarded the curled meeting of land and sea as sacred in their own peculiar way. The point was the whale itself, made of both land and sea. Iñupiat cosmology brought all objects into the same spirit universe as the living spirits of animals and humans. The land, the lagoons, and the sea were not regarded as forms independent of life; they had souls.

In my experience of other points, such as at Orfordness and Portland Bill in Britain, at Provincetown off Long Island, at Cape Hatteras in North Carolina, and at a peculiar point off the north of Cranberry Island, Maine, I have seen the same minigeography and experienced an uncanny spirit of place. ∎

Meanwhile, out in the sea we saw sea gulls with black wing tips, huge herring gulls, and cormorants, dipping and returning. Sandpipers were scurrying near the waves.

2

A Dream of the Loss of Childhood

September 9, Wednesday. We were able to eat elders' lunch more often because the schedule was changed to include every week day. This Wednesday Netta Jackson appeared at the lunch and sat down. So here was Netta again. I had been hearing controversial views of her. Who was she? I saw her as a small and slightly scary person, and I had heard she was a healer. I asked her permission to sit next to her, which she granted. We said grace silently. Then we ate breaded cube steak, corn, macaroni, french fries, and slaw, followed by a Jello-plus-CoolWhip dessert in styrofoam cups, which we were able to take home, everyone having been provided with cup lids.

I said, "I'm English, you know. Not American."

Netta commented, "It was the English who started the church in Ivakuk. They used to send a lot of free clothes to the village."

"Good. My own parents were Episcopalian," I said hopefully. But the conversation faded.

September 11, Friday. Things became difficult at Friday's elders' lunch. It leaked out that I had been sitting in on the ninth grade high school Iñupiat class, run by Helen Pingasut's brother, Ed. Netta asked if I paid the school for this.

"Not as far as I know."

"That's cheating the Iñupiat," said Netta.

Guilty on all counts!

I explained, "The Iñupiaq teacher gave me permission."

Evidently they thought of me as a White exploiter, me, a lifelong liberal. I knew who had been cheating the Iñupiat. The Alaska Native Claims Settlement Act of 1971 flashed into my mind.

"You're right," I said. "We Whites have been cheating the Iñupiat in a big way. I know what went on. Whites took your oil land, paid you less than three dollars an acre for it, then the Whites tied you up with lawyers for the land rights and the legalities of the payment, and afterward here in Ivukak another lot of con men did you out of the principal in a shady investment deal. Now they say that the agreement was that in 1991 all the land you have left could be sold to Whites—they could get the natives into debt and force the sale of your land, the only thing you have. That's their marvelous Alaska Native Claims Settlement Act of 1971.[1] Anything I can possibly do, I'm on your side."

There was silence. We finished our lunch.

I was even more determined to become acquainted with old Netta—a healer, after all. So, later that afternoon, greatly daring, Carrie and I found our way along the grid-pattern streets and knocked at her door. There was a hoarse yell of "Come in!"

We entered the porch, made our way past some squabbling small boys, and found ourselves in a capacious modern living room. We saw family photographs filling the walls, a couch against one wall, and at the other end of the room near the kitchen alcove a large table littered with cups and pilot bread, that is, large round crackers made of hardtack. The dining chairs had torn seats. On the side by the kitchen stood a clean garbage bin full of water in which floated one-foot chunks of ice; there was also a big refrigerator. In the kitchen alcove dirty dishes were piled in the sink. A huge TV stood in front of the couch, full on. Clem Jackson, Netta's middle-aged grandson, lay sprawled on the beat-up couch smoking a cigarette, watching the TV. He turned a large, wide-open face to me.

"Sit down." He rose and wiped off the table, then poured us cups of coffee.

"Thanks." The coffee cheered me up, so I started talking about the importance of subsistence. I tried not to ask incessant questions. I simply talked, to begin with.

"I've made an *umiak*," Clem told us. "I'll be a whaling captain this season."

"Have you ever ki—caught a whale?" (I realized I must not use the word *kill*.)

"No. But I have a crew now."

Carrie started on a new theme. "Do you make masks?" she said.

"Yes, faces of ivory." We leaned forward attentively. He continued speaking because we were willing to listen. "The mask is the whale's face. When the whale's parka is taken off you see the whale's face. It's a human face inside." The sentences were coming out with a quiet inevitability, singsong and particularized, Clem's eyes looking at us searchingly. I liked this. "When you catch a whale you give back its face to the sea: then the whale grows a new parka. It can only do it twice, not more than twice. After that the whale becomes another animal and the face is different." I immediately thought, "So this is the meaning of those bone and ivory faces displayed in Alaskan museums. They are the faces of the human spirits of the animals." [Before my trip north I had been trying to practice Native American shamanism myself and was interested in animal spirits.]

Carrie put in, "It's the same for the salmon among the Nootka and the Tlingit. Every bone must go back to the water." Carrie, for her part, was using her specialized knowledge of Indian culture. Her engagement to an Indian gave her some importance here.

A very old man entered the room with a shuffling step. He was extraordinarily short in stature. Netta, who came in with him, told us, "He's like a child now." Clem pointed out proudly that this old personage was his grandfather, and not only that, he was the great-grandfather of some of the little boys whom I had seen sparring in the passageway and the great-great-grandfather of some of the others. A small boy had a bruise by his eye. He came up to his great-grandmother and gave her his mitten, which was turned the wrong side out. She fixed it for him, peering at it from her little withered eyes, then did the same with the other mitten. Here was Netta in her ordinary low-pulse home environment.

September 13, Sunday.   Frosts began here and there. There was always so much wind. We had now learned to take the wind for granted as we wove in and out among the separated houses on our way to the store, always plodding against the loose pebbles with a forward-leaning motion, as everyone else did. [The women's parkas were ideal for life in Ivakuk. They were often made with a soft tuscany lamb lining an inch thick and had no buttons or zippers, so that one took them off by bending over and tossing them forward. The hood had a special Ivakuk cut with extra fullness around the nape of the neck to accommodate a baby. The hood was crowned with a magnificent wolverine ruff. These parkas were beautiful garments, custom made from gorgeously printed velveteen, lined and windproof, and ornamented with complex trimming at the low waist. The low waist gave one a low center of gravity, so that some-how the short frilled skirt below, tipped with peeping fur at the hem, seemed to have aerodynamic qualities—it frilled out and caused one to float along. A tubby woman like Dora Nashanik looked splendid, and obviously felt splendid, in her grand parka.]

That night I dreamed I was participating with the members of some conference or other, all of whom I knew—but when I awoke I didn't remember any of them. One seemed to "look like" Barbara Myerhoff, my dead friend, another was "like" Thelma Lupton, a person I knew in the fifties. We arrived in a conference bus at the front door of a big house, which was "like" my old home at Ely in England, long since demolished. In my dream we disembarked from the bus and entered the house. It was empty of furniture. We all slept on the floor in one room, as I had actually done a month earlier in a Zen temple in Korea, along with a similar party of con-ferees. I liked the place, and realized more and more how similar it was to my old home. I went into the big rooms. They corre-sponded to the old rooms, alike, yet not the same, just as the con-ference members were like my old friends but not the same. A pas-sage going through the house to the back led out to the garden. The back door was in the same position as the back door of long ago; also there were windows vaguely similar to those of my fa-ther's consulting room. He had been a medical doctor. In my dream, on the right, where the greenhouse used to be, stood a shed. The grass was thick and green; the lawn was smaller than the old one, and on the far side of the lawn stood a big round tree, closely resembling the old chestnut tree of my youth, a tree that held great significance for me because as children we used to climb it. A large, low horizontal branch used to extend from the trunk, on which we had once tied a swing, and here it was again. In the dream I was rather amazed at these similarities, thinking, "Of course this isn't a dream, it's real, but it might have been a dream." I was vaguely aware of a manuscript I had been writing, in which I had discussed different levels of consciousness, and wondered if I had penetrated to a different level of consciousness now.

Still continuing in the dream, I went back into the house, dawdling about although I knew the bus would leave pretty soon. And sure enough, when I regained the front of the house, the bus had gone, leaving no one around. What was worse, outside in front of the house it was pouring with rain, dark, solid, perma-nent-looking rain. I felt that I would never be able to hitch a ride in the rain. Then I had an idea that I was in my sleeping bag, and

sure enough I was, I was in Ivakuk. I was greatly relieved to find
that I wasn't stranded after all but was safe in my bed.

Long afterward I thought about this dream. Here were
three transformations: old faces and my old home, with a
sense of it all being "like" this and that, and yet not alike,
and always the sense that it was not a dream. Something
had slipped. The house and garden were empty. Did I have the
sense long ago in the garden that a future me was looking back at
this scene? Did I even then have a feeling of this estrangement,
possibly fed in from the future strangeness of Ivakuk but now
warning me that the past was canceled? This cancellation took place
in the second transformation, the rain, the situation of being cut off
from the others and stranded, with no way out but actual reality;
and that final realization was the third stage, the reality of Ivakuk.
And in my dream I had been writing about different levels of consciousness. This actual book, *The Hands Feel It,* was developing levels of the same sort. I meant to let them enter the narrative wherever they had to enter. ∎

But at that time in Ivakuk I needed to hold tight to ordinary reality, and I decided to look at the politics of the village.

September 15, Tuesday.   The politics were mainly centered
on the Ivakuk Native Corporation office, the headquarters of the
Iñupiat tribal business corporation of which the store and motel
were part. The office was a prefab, like all the houses, only larger.
In the entrance hall I saw displayed on the wall some large aerial
photographs of the village, set some way down from the point of
the land, also a superb architect's conception of the investment deal
I had mentioned at the elders' lunch [this was an office block in
Anchorage that was never actually built. Where had the funds
gone? I wondered.]

At one of the native corporation desks sat Micky Hoffman, an
Iñupiaq intellectual with a sparse, protruding beard and anxious
eyes. This man was the people's advocate against the White legal
system. [White law seemed to have gained some control over the
failing village corporation and might take it over altogether if it
weakened further. As it was, a White judge was legal monitor of the
corporation while it remained in Chapter 11. The native corporation employed Micky because he was training himself as a lawyer.
He was their expert.]

Micky was an uneasy man. He sat turning the pages of an official

letter while we talked. "Did you know that Ivakuk is built over Iñupiat graves on the southeastern corner?" he volunteered.

"Was it?" I was shocked. "Did the people here make that decision? Surely not."

"Yes, they did. When we had to move, the corporation members
made the decision, in fact they passed the town planning officer's
plans; but they were misinformed. They were misinformed," he repeated thoughtfully. "There were consequences," he went on, lowering his voice on "consequences." His voice began to vibrate a little. "People went mad in one of the houses and had to leave. The
next family that took over the house went mad too. Near one site
there was a telegraph pole, a big one. It was snapped clean off.
Funny things were seen. . . . I've been trying to correct it," he said
leaning back. "But . . ." ("What funny things were seen?" I wondered. "Anything like Edwina's Hook Man?")

He went on, "There's supposed to be a meeting about it this afternoon at five. I don't see anybody coming." He looked mournful
and stroked his beard.

"Is there anything I can do to help?"

"Write a letter. What is most important is to write about our
land rights here in Ivakuk, and send it to our northern newspaper."

"OK. I'll come and discuss it pretty soon."

[After some discussion I composed a letter. In it I raised issues
about the serious matter of the people's lack of legal title to their
village land. During the year that followed, the Iñupiat's pressure
for title continued, culminating in allotment papers being issued.
My letter was but a fraction of all the efforts being made. The letter
had a side effect, though, for I believe it bore certain unpleasant
consequences for me at Bristol (see chapter 6).]

While I was sitting with Micky, Netta Jackson entered and went
past Micky's desk to the Ivakuk Native Corporation office, the
INC.

"What are you at?" asked Micky.

"It's my birthday tomorrow," she said in her quavering voice. "I
need cake mix and eggs for the cake, and I'm out of cash. I'll get
the IC to lend me some." The IC was Ivakuk Corporation. She
bustled in to the IC manager's inner office. She remained there for
quite a while, being a determined old lady. I was beginning to respect her.

Back she came. "Well?" said Micky.

"No good." And she toddled off home. After finishing with
Micky I went off to a private store and purchased six eggs and half

a pound of butter, then stumbled off myself over the gravel to Netta's house and delivered the groceries.

September 17, Thursday. Two days later—careful to wait until after the party because we hadn't been invited—Carrie and I visited Netta. After we knocked, we heard her bustling about inside. When we recognized her shrill "Come in!" we made our way past the crowding parkas hung in the passageway and immediately saw that Netta had been busy arranging the old man in an armchair with a blanket over his lap. This old husband of hers had Alzheimer's disease, and nursing him was proving a difficult task.

Netta was happy to tell us all about the birthday party, how they ate caribou, frozen fish, and birthday cake. It had been a big party, for it was her seventy-eighth birthday; she was the head of a great family of Jacksons, 75 of them in a village of 660 persons. Carrie gave the old lady a necklace made of what she called "whitehearts," red beads with white hearts, highly valued by Native Americans. Clem's wife handed around home-made bread and butter and coffee.

I ventured on the topic of storytelling with Netta.

"Those stories," she said. "I've told them in books. You'll find them."

"I wonder what it was like when you were young."

"I remember it. I remember being six years old. That was when my grandmother died. I lay on her chest and wouldn't get off. My mother was crying, but I wasn't crying." Netta leaned over to me and said. "I remember when I was born." This woman was a healer and probably had always possessed a remarkable kind of consciousness.

"You must have remembered the shamans."

She shuddered. "Them. They killed my babies." Then her tone changed. "When I was eight they healed me of my stomach trouble. For years I had been getting thinner and thinner, and I nearly died." Netta looked at me, remembering. "My Aunt Judy was the shaman. She felt all over my stomach and trunk and found that my stomach was up. She put my stomach back in its right position, then took the trouble in her hands." Netta cupped her own hands half an inch apart, then raised her hands, blew into them, "And she blew the trouble up out of the smoke hole." There was a ventilator in the ceiling of her house, and she blew toward that.

"Yes, the shamans delivered babies. Suellen, my niece, works on people—I taught her." Suellen was famous in the north for her healing.

I told myself that I would have to get used to these curious oscillations from bad memories of shamanism to good, from fear to blissful wonder. I bent to hear.

"—And the giant bird, *tingmiaqpak*," she was saying. "They saw it, the men saw it. My brother-in-law and my Uncle Runiq were out toward the southern sea cliffs. There it was, with feet as high as you, and wings as wide as this room." Netta looked from end to end of the room. Her voice was quavering but authoritative. "The men went to one side of it. It flew up heavily. They shot it under the wing pit." Netta pointed dramatically to her armpit. "It flew away."[2] [I heard elsewhere it so frightened the men that they gave up hunting for weeks.]

The conversation changed. Clem Jackson proudly indicated the speechless old man sitting with the rug on his lap. "My grandfather won land rights for Ivakuk. He was the greatest dancer in the village, and he worked in the corporation and the post office. He won 'Historic Site' status for the entire beach as far as the southern cape. That law is now hard and fast. The status includes the people because they have been there all along. For many thousands of years," he added quietly. "So legally the people can't be touched. I've applied to be curator of this historic site." [But I discovered that the Alaskan Whites took no notice of this law, coming as it did under federal law, not state law. Oil, not history, was king in the state.]

Clem talked politics. He was brilliant in the language of bureaucracy and lost me time after time. He described the suppression of shamanism, the subtle pressures from the Whites to assimilate, and the way the oil lands were appropriated. "It was easy to take the good grace of our people," he said, sighing.

I left the Jacksons to go to the language class at the high school, where I encountered a sparse showing of ninth to twelfth graders. The teacher's Iñupiaq aide was giving the students the names of the arctic villages of the North Slope. She pointed to one village on the map. "You're supposed to spell it 'Anaktuv*uk*,'" she said.

"It should be 'vik,' which means place," said Edwin Tukumavik, the teacher's son, also the brother of Edwina.

"Yes, it's wrong," she said sadly. "But we have to spell it as they do on the map, and the map isn't right."

"We have no rights," muttered young Tommie. "We won't have any in 1991—we'll have no land."

"We were born after 1971, so we don't have any land anyway," said Edwin. He turned around to Dick Kuper at the back and said, "What are you going to do when you grow up, Dick?"

"Join the *army!*" said Dick with horrid irony. "Have my head shaved all around the back." He passed his hand savagely around the back of his thick black hair.

I muttered, "Don't stand for it, kids. Do something about it." I loved them. They resisted education, yet they were extremely intelligent.

These first weeks gradually revealed an ever moving picture of an ebullient, family-linked community that rather liked itself—a community of people who were always telling stories, that is, to those to whom the stories carried the power they contained (Goulet 1994). Carrie and I had already walked to the end of the beach, had seen a little snow in early September, and had become interested in the warm coats of the Iñupiat. We had picked up scraps of odd lore about the whale, but as yet we saw no sign of whaling except for some tourist art in the Ivakuk Native Corporation office showroom, a jawbone outside the house of an old man called Kagliq, and the bones at the cemetery. We had noted the physical strength and short stature of the people, their irrepressible tendency to laugh, their restraint and watchfulness, and the burning though suppressed politics. Here was Clem, doing my fieldwork for me, explaining the Ivakuk view of the animals. I was beginning to think about the words of Ann Fienup-Riordan, who well understood the Yup'ik Eskimo sense of cosmological cycling. In her book *The Nelson Island Eskimos* (1983), she explains how seals' bladders are thrown back into the sea to regrow a new seal, and how the whole universe similarly turns on its circle and replaces itself in the cycling of the cosmos. Clem was explaining the same thing. This time I was not reading about the principle in a book. Among my new acquaintances the whale did reincarnate, and that was that. Was this the same as the idea of a renewable universe? Was it the same as Charles Kingsley's scene of the remaking of the animals in *The Water Babies* (1928), a book that featured a majestic female figure far in the north who says of the animals that come to her to die, and are sent out from her renewed, "I make them make themselves." That book was a novel, but it was oddly predictive of concepts explored by environmentalists more than a century later.

Nearby at the ancient graves, Kaglik and Claire's grandfather-in-law, cooperating with archeologists, had found animal carvings depicting the same kinds of souls that Clem had mentioned as dwelling within the animals. The ideas were old and recurred in much of North American native religion and art, and all around the arctic. ∎

September 19, Saturday. Looking along the shore, I glimpsed snow on the southern cape. The beautiful long peninsula of the northern cape was also visible on the opposite horizon, far beyond the lagoon. As I stood out on the shore, I saw many things: a boat on the southern sea, a plane arriving, a truck proceeding along the lagoon shore, five Honda all-terrain vehicles (ATVs) here and there, two dogs, many arctic squirrels standing up and threatening me, a seagull. A big black raven was sitting on a rack that held a polar bear skin spread out to dry. The raven flew away, "*Kark!*" It was a bird that commanded respect. There was another seagull. All was totally quiet now except for an almost imperceptible booming. It was the ice behind me on the lagoon. Right here tiny plants melted themselves into visibility and got chewed by the squirrels for their pains. Everywhere around us could be seen twenty-foot-wide masses of grass tufts, each mass an old sod house. I counted ninety of them as I walked. I could see the sod still banked up around one of them.

September 20, Sunday. After that quiet Saturday, Sunday came like a flooding-in of spirit experience, like a dream. The church was empty when I entered—it was rather fine, walled with pale oak mass-produced paneling. I poked into the vestry and caught sight of red choir vestments arranged on hangers, and a box of matches on a window sill, hinting of candles. I walked slowly back to the body of the church and turned. On the wall above the altar glimmered a scene from the Gospels. Now in front of me appeared a young black-haired acolyte clothed in a red cassock. He was lighting the candles on the high altar. He looked beautiful holding his long brass candle lighter; he extinguished the flame in the lighter when he was done, then moved away backward until he was down the altar step, then a moment of respect, then to the next step, a turn, another moment of respect, then he went away.

The service was beginning. Choir men and women took their places, and a serious Iñupiaq preacher entered, short in stature, round of face, wearing a white surplice and stole. During the service he sometimes spoke in Iñupiat, sometimes in English. During the hymns I noticed Seth Lowe, a grizzled whaling captain, sitting behind me. I could hear him sing a hearty bass, and many women were singing alto, so I sang tenor, and we harmonized quite well. "Stand up, stand up for Jesus / Ye soldiers of the cross" was one hymn. The theme running through the service was battle, death, human weakness, the desire for suicide, and God's triumph. The reading was from Jonah and the whale. Tears did not seem very far from any of us. I noticed the tears of others through my blur. [I did not know it then, but Ivakuk was combining for me all the warmth of my large family with the separation from home I suffered as a tiny child at boarding school—situated as it was on a spit of land in the North Sea, England. I could not believe that I should be liked and protected in such a place, instead of being teased and bullied. Yet it was so.]

As the service went on, I could see it was snowing slightly outside. Those inside wore their finest parkas; they were mostly my elders' lunch crowd, along with a few young families. After it was over, the preacher shook hands with everybody, and the congregation took off smartly into the cold weather, some on Honda three-wheelers.

September 21, Monday.   Back to politics. This morning I succeeded at last in mailing the letter to the newspaper about Iñupiat rights and the people's concerns over the land issue. [The letter was published.]

3
The Healer

September 21, Monday. Now I took my courage in both hands and went to visit the healer Claire Sivuq. While I was walking across the gravel to see Claire, I was wondering, wasn't she going to be secretive and reserved as Native Americans are said to be? My steps crunched the gravel beside a closely-built row of prefabricated houses. I was at the far side of the rectangular village, facing the mountains. At last Claire's house stood before me, painted dark red, with wooden steps going up from the gravel toward a door on the left. I ascended and knocked. Would she be at home?

A distant voice hollered, "Come in!" I opened the door. It was pitch dark inside. Ah, there was another door beyond: this was just 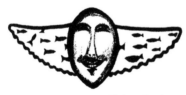 the storm porch. Shutting the first door against the bitter September wind, I opened the further one and found myself in a large living room.

Claire had just arrived back from a three-day healing trip in Bristol. She disappeared to change her clothes, so while I waited for her I looked around. Her living room was homey. There was a mop across the sofa. Photographs crowded the walls, as in my mother's old bedroom—especially a large color picture of Claire's mother-in-law Joanna Sivuq wearing a fur ruff. Joanna's thrawn yet cheerful features were ugly-beautiful, forming a picture in brown and gold. Another picture showed the Sivuq whaling crew busy on an enormous whale, with cuts already made in its side. Near Joanna's photograph was the famous picture of Jesus by Sallman, painted by the artist from a vision—the Savior's face burningly divine and all-knowing. Near it was the usual large clock. I saw a sewing machine in its table, and an Eddie Bauer man's down jacket waiting for repairs with the zipper tacked into place. A milk crate stood by the wall, containing neat files holding easily available forms. This constituted the village food stamp system, of which Claire was the organizer. Claire evidently ran things well. There were no photos anywhere of Claire herself.

The woman who entered the room seemed slightly distracted. The face looking at me was oval, serious, with fine, long features. There was an unusual attentiveness in it. Yes, she was interested in people and their bodies. She was somewhat like the dark-haired sibyl in Michelangelo's Sistine frescoes, but without the expression of terror, and carrying in her eyes the more delicate epicanthic structure of the Native American. I introduced myself to this healer person, thinking, "Come on, Edie, your own dad was a doctor. You're fascinated by healing for what it is. You've seen a thing or two." This woman possessed a gift, and I was ready and open to hear about it.

She knew that I was ready as we sat down.

I started out, "I've heard of your work. I've a great respect for Iñupiat healing."

"What made you interested in it?" she asked.

I told her the most dramatic healing event I knew. "I once saw my husband Vic heal somebody. This man had a heart attack in our living room and his heart stopped. Vic put his hand on the man's heart, and it started again. I still wonder what was going on—if I might learn what's behind it. I've a lot of respect for what you do."

"*I'm very glad.* I've been getting discouraged, frustrated." She looked away.

"Are the medical doctors getting you down?"

"Yes."

"Don't let 'em," I said. "It's a good work you're doing."

She and I liked each other. Her adopted children crowded around, Jeanie and Ann. She also had four other adopted children and two grandchildren. We began to talk about our families and grandchildren.

Claire said, "The baby, Jeanie, she's seven. Jeanie wants to be a healer like me. The kid's learning it already." She looked at Jeanie with appreciation. Then she was silent, pondering a minute. "Iñupiat healing is *different*." She lingered over the word. "Come into the kitchen and talk while I work."

In a few minutes she was due to attend a five o'clock teleconference education class and needed to hurry. She was taking anthropology. "Anthropology?" I thought. "She could *teach* them that, couldn't she?" So she had to go out right now. She had just come back from a trip and now she had to go out again. The kitchen was high with dirty dishes—the family had not washed them all the time she had been away. She was worried about the time, and about her children. She turned sharply to Ann. "What math homework do you have?" she spat. Ann showed her the book.

"You can do that quickly. Do the dishwashing, then the homework."

"I'll do the dishwashing," I said, and got to work. It was easy because there was plenty of hot running water. Just as I started, a message came over Claire's CB radio. She cocked an ear.

"Claire, come on in. Claire, come on in," the voice said. "Go to Netta's at once; she's sick. She's throwing up." The anthropology class would have to be missed because Netta, an elder, was sick, and healing always came first. Before leaving, Claire thought for a moment, then went to her refrigerator. In it stood two jars of a blackish fluid, made from the best of the Iñupiat herbs, *qanganaruaq,* called stinkweed. [This is actually a fragrant plant classified as *Artemisia tilesii,* wormwood—also related to a traditional medicine of Europe, absinthe. It is cousin to our popular plant dusty miller and smells like chamomile.] Claire took out some of the boiled infusion and drank a cupful to give her healing strength; she handed me a little to try myself. It was bitter and heartening. Claire grabbed her coat and left. I left also, after finishing the dishes, and went home for a bite to eat. There I began to think: "A healing's in progress," and decided that I too would go to Netta's house.

As I approached Netta's door, a woman came out. She passed me and jumped on her Honda ATV.

"How is she?" I asked.

"Netta plays too much bingo," she said. "So of course she doesn't eat properly. That's why she's sick." This was the head of the health aides in the clinic. I went inside.

There were many people in Netta's living room. I went along the passage to Netta's bedroom and found Clem at the entrance of the room. His flat face was loosened into solemnity, unseeing. I peeped into the room. Netta was lying on a mattress on the floor, not on her bed. She was clothed in a skirt and a fine blouse, with white tube socks on her feet. Claire was at her side with Jeanie, her seven-year-old healing apprentice, sitting between her knees. My friend Carrie had already found her way there and was helping. Above Netta's head I could see another copy of Sallman's Jesus, set up against the window frame, along with an open Bible.

The old man was sitting on the unoccupied bed. He arose and stood near, then went wandering off down the passage. After a time back he came again, and this went on all the while—the old man shuffling to and fro, to and fro. Ardell Lowe, another health aide, was sitting on the bed, backstage, as it were, to Claire. Carrie told me Netta's stomach was in the wrong position, and it was hard and tight. Claire could feel air pockets that were stopping the stomach from working, causing Netta to vomit blood. Netta hadn't been able to eat for three days.

When I returned to the living room, I realized how many people had gathered in the moment of old Netta's danger: close kin, cousins, nieces, and many grown-up grandchildren. I greeted the elders. These were Kaglik, who was Netta's brother, with high cheekbones and eyes downcast, and Netta's son, Clem's father. Both of them were old men. They sat like statues on straight chairs. There was silence. I felt a little frightened. Then I went back to Netta, and Carrie and I took to massaging Netta's feet to relax her. But she vomited, groaning, and lay back; then she vomited again and muttered something in Iñupiat. The healer, Claire, was working on Netta's stomach with both hands, working deep into the folds of the old stomach flesh. Claire had "good hands," as the Iñupiat often said: those hands could soothe and take away pain. At one point Claire spread out both arms with her fingers wide in a gesture of relief. She was tired. In Iñupiat parlance Netta's stomach had risen and was jammed against her heart and lungs, stopping those organs from functioning properly. I went to Ardell, the health aide. "What's wrong, d'you think?"

"We don't know. I'm going to have to phone the hospital and get them to send the medevac plane. The senior health aide gave Netta some Mylanta. That's all we are allowed to do."

Claire, meanwhile, was softening Netta's stomach to bring it down into the right position. But the air pocket gave trouble. Standing now in the doorway, I saw the old woman's face become contorted, then I saw it blank out to nothing. Claire held Netta's head hard and held on, holding Netta to her. I started to pray. Clem looked fearful, as if death impended; perhaps it did. The old lady reared up again in agony to vomit, then fell back. Her body blanked out and her head sank back. She looked emptied. Claire massaged her stomach, bending her head very near to Netta's head. Once Claire put her hands on Netta's stomach and lay her head upon her hands, right on the stomach.

Ardell, the health aide, watched, then betook herself off to the clinic to make the phone call to the hospital at Bristol. I went off for some snacks and brought them back to feed Claire and the others. I looked at the scene through the door and saw the lax figure and the supporting forms, Claire's leaning care, Carrie at the feet: "Oh Netta, I'm sad for your pain, sad." And I turned to the Iñupiat way myself, trying to remember how it must have been. The healer makes his journey to find the lost spirit of the sick person. Netta's spirit? And what kind of being was that? You go down a tunnel, and you try to find Netta's animal. It would be her helping spirit. Standing at the entrance of the bedroom I tried it. A tunnel. And there appeared a polar bear. The beast wouldn't go away and seemed to hover softly around—which was odd, with the jostle nearby and little boys whizzing toy cars down the passage. Again! I saw the jaws of the bear. I might be swallowed. Okay, let me be swallowed, and so I was. Inside the animal and yet grasping it, I turned, drawing the whole of it with me. The thing to do was to go quickly back through the tunnel. I was through. Now I had to look with ordinary eyes at the ordinary world around me. I had to give that animal to Netta. From behind the people I made a small flute mouth and blew the animal to her, then blew again, hard, straight, and long. She stirred to vomit. I blew once more, letting go all of it. She lay back. And who could tell? I was also praying that Claire would heal her. Everyone involved has to do all she knows how. Netta lay there exhausted; was she failing or resting? Claire stayed right close to her, head to head, with her hand always on Netta's stomach, warmly there with the "different" knowledge in it, an intimate contact. I thought, "If only they had done that for me when I was in the hospital in 1983 for agonizing stomach cramps."

Netta stayed as she was, still vomiting occasionally. Each time she vomited we looked anxiously at the clock wondering when the plane would come. But she did seem to be resting. Claire began to talk cheerfully. I loved Claire's ordinary conversation—this was some gossip about her grown-up son and his new TV. We laughed, subduing our voices. The others all talked in Iñupiat. Netta was now drinking Seven Up, talking, and complaining vividly in Iñupiat about her stomach. She stretched out her feet, which had been reincased in her tube socks. The old man entered the room in his tortoise crawl and stopped at her outstretched legs. He just managed to walk across them and go to sit on the bed.

Netta asked for some tea. There was a quiet rush to fetch her a cup. Clem began to smile. Another healer, Pamela, took over from Claire for a while. Gradually we became aware that the immediate crisis was past. Carrie went to the kitchen and washed the dishes along with Clem's wife, Margie. We waited.

The plane was flying over. Everyone heard it. The people in the living room, dressed in their grand velveteen parkas and huge ruffs, passed to and fro to look through the windows, telling each other, "There it is." Clem started worrying about intravenous feeding, IVs—"She must have fluids. The doctor will have to do the IV in the house; the ambulance is too small." Margie fussed over what clothes to send with her. Even so, they forgot her dentures.

As we stood waiting, Clem said to me in his slow voice: "Her spirit went out of her body three times. Three times it went out of her, and Claire brought it back and pulled it down into her stomach. A spirit—when it leaves it goes up through the hole in the top of the head." I touched my long-closed fontanel (the site of some of my headaches—a place that was aching a little that day).

Clem said, "That's right, there."

Claire's healing acts of drawing back the spirit were the same as the ancient Iñupiat shamanic healings that used to be performed in the old sod houses at the end of the point. But this occasion was *now*.

I stood with Clem, still frightened for Netta's safety, finding I was already dominated by love for the old lady and for this crowd that had become my "forever" acquaintances. "Forever"? After three weeks? I was getting involved.

There was a stir. The ambulance had arrived, a new yellow low-slung vehicle that had been backed up just by the door. Marvin, the White pilot, came in; then a tall, dark-haired, White man, distant of manner, who turned out to be the doctor; another bearded little fellow, quite fun; then a huge White ambulance man, easy to talk to. The place was full of people milling around in a confused way. I peered into Netta's room. A White nurse was already there, putting a blood pressure sleeve on Netta's arm. This nurse knew the Jacksons from Margie's recent childbirth visit to the hospital. The team became occupied in following the stereotypes of medical practice. They took the blood pressure, pulse, and temperature, and asked questions, and then the stretcher men gathered in the bedroom.

Clem went and told the doctor, "She's been spitting out very dark stuff, black, like blood." The doctor came up the passage to the bedroom and looked into the old lady's vomiting can. "A little blood," he said disparagingly. I returned to the living room, and the doctor came and stood by the wall. We grew silent. After a moment the ambulance men emerged from the passageway with their stretcher—Netta was in it. They carried her out the door and into the ambulance. We saw her wrinkled face lifted to look out of the ambulance, then the doors were shut, and they were off to the air strip.

Here I depart from the strict calendar and relate later events that completed this episode. The news came through little by little from the Anchorage hospital, and it varied. Netta had not yet been diagnosed, she had had an operation, she had not had an operation, they had removed a cyst from her as big as a baby, she had not yet had an X-ray, she had nearly died in the airplane, she had needed oxygen all the way, she was better, she was very weak, and her dentures were left behind—which amused everybody.

After several weeks I saw her restored and back in her living room, her little proud head wobbling a bit and her halting words begging me to work on her stomach because of the wind. Very softly I did, and tried to pray as the healers did. Then I cooked her some cream of wheat because she was hungry.

She had indeed had a huge cyst removed—"as big as a baby"— and after the operation she gradually regained her active, combative temperament. ∎

September 24, Thursday.   Carrie and I visited Claire at 11:15 A.M. We found her living room crammed with five large plastic laundry hampers full of dirty washing, and the couch piled high with clothes. Claire was cooking bacon and eggs for Zeke, her husband, who was a big man in the village, a whaling captain, and was employed by the Borough Construction Unit to build snowmobile garages for the corporation houses, starting with his own. Claire said, "Have some coffee"—then dashed to the utility room, where an old but efficient agitator washer was working, now in the cycle of agitating a full load of men's jeans that were swilling about in some already used rinsing water. The washer was topped with a built-in electric wringer. Claire wrung the jeans. We helped her turn them inside out afterward, and she put them through again. We helped with much of the washing, hung up the jeans on the overhead pipes, swept the floor of the living room, and folded the clothes piled on the sofa, while she talked and worked alongside us. She was describing the sense that she had of feeling the pain of the sick.

"I can feel the sick person's pain; I can feel where it is. Do you get how I mean? A woman in a village 250 miles away called me and said, 'I'm having a miscarriage.' She was four months pregnant. When the woman spoke, I knew what was wrong—it's my second sight. My second sight told me how to advise the woman. I told her what to do. The fetus was saved and the baby was born full term."

Claire said again, "My healing is *different*. The doctors say, 'You're wrong, Claire.' They think I'm trying to do predictions—I don't predict, I *know* when someone's pregnant and for how long. Then it turns out I'm right. The health aides say 'You must go by what the doctors say'—but I *know*. They finished my employment at the clinic, I don't know why. One woman came to me. She put out her hand and said, 'Don't touch me.'" Claire put out her hand and drew it back. "I didn't touch her. I told her she was two weeks pregnant. I *knew*. In a month she took the test, and she was pregnant. She was scared."

"Why should people be scared of what is good and useful?" I asked.

Claire went to do more laundry. There she was slaving for her family, washing, waiting on them with food and services.

"I'm glad you came. For thirty years no one's helped me in the house," she said. She picked up a glittering peacock blue velvety bathrobe, wet from the washtub. "I made this myself, for Zeke," she said proudly. Zeke was in the back bedroom watching TV. She went in there later to hang up the nicer things, knitted sweaters and so on. I was thinking how her healing gifts ought to be backed up.

Claire talked a blue streak. She said to Carrie and me, "You and Edie are different." That was odd. Just two hours earlier Carrie and I had been talking about that difference, trying to define our difference from other Whites. I looked at Carrie and she looked back.

I told Claire about Philip Kabwita, the African healer, who had received a message by spirit telephone from 350 miles away;[1] then I talked about Netta's illness.

"If you hadn't been there when Netta was sick she might have died," I said.

"I saw the spirit leaving her several times," said Claire. "Her stomach was blocked. I had to be there. What would Netta have done without any help?"

"She'd have died," I said.

Portrait of Claire. I remember Claire, with the oval face and high forehead. She looks out from herself, all alive, with a considering expression in her eyes. Claire moves with an easy walk and big, fluid motions. She takes her jacket off in my house and sits down, ready for anything, with her eyes a little hooded as becomes an Iñupiaq (it is rude to look straight into a person's eyes), yet watchful and confident. She is capable and looks after herself; she asks for what does not appear on the table, such as honey to put in her tea. Her voice wanders into great variations in tone, rasping (during the telling of an uncertainty) along with a note of self-assertion, sometimes slumping in falling tones, changing to complaint, still in rasp. But when she muses or reminisces, her voice is wandering and soft, musically keyed, her eyes inward, her mind seeing pictures that leap into existence one on top of the other—the voice leaps as the memories come. And when she is teaching me language pronunciation,[2] then she lets out sounds full of the most sorrowful rasping, and searching, and persisting, and she is near to despair, with a frog in her throat and much doubt, then a ray of hope. She tries me again with *qa-aɲɲaq*, "rough." I repeat, "kargak," incorrectly, and her hands flop uselessly by her side. She laughs—cackles like the grandmother she is.

I know a certain thing about her from long ago and cannot bear to think about it. It was when she stood before her burning house with her first three children dying inside it, her spirit dead and tortured within her. A screaming impossibility, Claire.

Now with six children more, adopted, and three grandchildren, with an easy job she likes, sitting in City Hall, typing on a computer, running the teleconferences—that is the life (only they recently cut down her hours). And she has a telephone and a CB, so she is in a position to answer sickness calls.

Claire's life, impelled by the high tragedy long ago, passes through chambers and histories beyond mere words. Where I attempt words, they come best in their own time, in context.

During Claire's treatment of Netta, four of us—Claire, Clem, Carrie, and to a certain extent, I—could perceive how Netta's spirit continually parted company with her tortured organs and wandered toward its outlet in her fontanel. Claire freed the blockage in the stomach again and again and brought the spirit back down into Netta's body. The activity of Claire's arms and head showed what she was doing.

Normally, when the blood flows well, and when the stomach and organs are in tune, well disposed, well aligned, well positioned, they are able to contain the spirit and maintain it happily. Iñupiat medical ideas clearly go beyond the physical boundaries of Western medical science and have no trouble with those boundaries. The Iñupiat healers do not diagnose an abstract concept called stress. Iñupiat knowledge has always existed athwart the boundaries of the levels of consciousness, just as the hunter's element is from ice floe to water, water to floe, and for that matter, in any place in the region.

Position, space, place, toward, those are concepts around which the Iñupiat language has developed 312 demonstrative adverbs, variants on *here* and *there* (MacClean 1980, 154–60), with obvious advantages to the hunter. The whole of life is looked upon in this *hither-and-thither* style. "Are you just staying at home?" comes the Iñupiat query. They are up and about, whizzing by on Hondas, twanging the tensions between siblings-in-law (one of many kinds of tension), and then at night setting ear to the sound of the wooden drumstick, called "striker," played sharply upon the far side of the wooden rim, only slightly touching the drum skin membrane or indirectly vibrating it. The striker whacks *across* the drum. Thereupon one hears two different sounds: the clack on the rim, *noise,* and the boom of the skin, *sonority.* Two things are done with the hands: there is a *near* and a reaching to something *beyond,* the one hand holding the drum handle firm, the other moving.

Not only is this dual activity a picture of Iñupiat awareness of levels of consciousness, but it may be compared to what the two hands do in healing, as well. The left hand holds the healthy organs in position while the right hand manipulates the displaced organ until it is correctly aligned and in its right position. Claire showed me how Iñupiat hands actually feel the difference between dead or sick tissue and what is alive and healthy. The healers at their tasks often put their hands on the opposite member of the patient's body, that which is healthy, so that they can more easily sense how the sick one is different. Then the hands know which part should be brought into its right place, what the sickness is. One hand holds firm, the other bridges the gulf. Because the hands know what dead or sick tissue feels like, the live is empowered, and the hands restore the communication. The bridging, in a sense, enters another level and has to do with the cycling of the cosmos (see Fienup-Riordan 1983)—runs with it. It has to do with spirit communication and, indirectly, even with reincarnation.

From that time on I was deluged with reports of healings, past and present. I observed many and participated in some of them myself. ∎

4
Embattled Politics

The Ancient Master Returns

September 29, Tuesday. Margie Jackson, Clem's wife, was from the Yup'iit, a people of western Alaska, not the Iñupiat. She was sometimes able to see things from the outside looking in. Yet she was married into the heart of Ivakuk. Both she and Clem had been married before to different partners, and a number of children had been born from both unions, some adopted in, some adopted out. Margie was going through a bad time with her new baby. When I entered her house she looked tired and had obviously been crying. I saw a thin, pale, weepy woman. She had eaten no breakfast, and her new baby hadn't fed much, though to me the baby

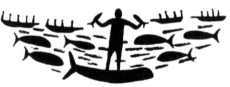

looked fine. I tried to cheer Margie up and get her to eat.

"Where's Clem?" I asked, when things had settled down.

"At the IRA meeting." I had learned that the IRA was the Indian Reorganization Act body in Ivakuk, also called the Native Village, or Tribal Government. "Clem says what he thinks at the IRA meetings," said Margie proudly.

Clem was known to be what I would call a patriot. "Nationalist" did not express what he was. The IRA was the only village power group the Iñupiat trusted. The people ran the meetings themselves, and its power stemmed directly from the federal government, not the state. Through it the land, the subsistence hunting, and minerals were guaranteed as the Iñupiat's own, their birthright in perpetuity, overriding any state laws.

It appeared that at the IRA meeting the members had been discussing land, a matter of perennial anxiety. The fruits of that discussion were going to be implemented at a meeting of the Ivakuk Native Corporation (INC), the village financial power body, on September 30, the coming morning. Native corporations had been set up in all the villages of native Alaska to control and invest the moneys stemming from the Alaska Native Claims Settlement Act of 1971. This corporation, like a number of others in Alaska, was in Chapter 11. ∎

Clem and his brother told me that the INC meeting would be open to the public, so I resolved to go along. I wanted to see how the power lines lay.

September 30, Wednesday. The door was locked at the corporation offices when I arrived. Eventually the village coordinator appeared, along with Norman Agnasagga, this year's chairman, and after them the other members. I noted the names and positions around the conference table. Micky Hoffman was there, with his nervous eyes; Claire's adopted son Rod, an employee of the INC, was there (he also represented the school board); and three revered old Iñupiat showed up, one of them being Sam, the tubby husband of my neighbor Annie Kasugaq, who had given me the fish. So there were seven Iñupiat men around the table. I saw one White man sitting at the side near the door, and there were also four women, including me, all of whom sat back by the wall, not around the table. Elana Lowe, the Iñupiaq store supervisor, sat in the inside corner along with Jenny, Margie's sister, who was the corporation secretary; I was in a chair backed off beside the wall near the door; and almost in the doorway itself sat a diminutive White woman lawyer. I was the only member of the public; everyone else in the conference room except North Slope Borough officials held a position on the INC. They looked me over as they came in but didn't seem to think I would do any harm. Indeed, I didn't speak during the proceedings.

At last they started with the meeting. The lawyer woman turned out to have some steel machinery in word form up her sleeve, but the picture was at first a blank to me.

The lawyer woman made the initial statement. She was a lawyer representing Legal Services. She was very "nice." She told the meeting that she was registering adoptions, and that if adoptive parents would agree to registration, their adoptive children would inherit their property. ("What could be more sensible?" I thought. And wondered.) The idea was that the Iñupiat had a right to enter the legal as well as the economic world of the Whites. "Do it. You'll benefit," she was saying. The assembly listened politely, the mature faces showing no feeling. I was aware that the Iñupiat people had developed an adoption system from ages back; adoptive children became their own children; it was simple. Under the hardships of polar conditions, easy adoption, especially by a grandmother, meant survival for the children when a parent happened to succumb to accident or starvation. An adopted child still had links with his or her old family, and these links became part of a system that fed into the complex web of connection that went around the village—a truly organic connection. This White lawyer meant only good, of course. She was nevertheless an agent of assimilation, codifying what did not need to be codified and paving the way with this and other such acts for the parceling out of every bit of land of the old free hunting territories.

No motion was made on the matter, and the lawyer retired from the room.

The White man near the door turned out to be an unusually tall man named Bruce Clay. In other contexts he would have seemed of average height, but I was now getting used to the height of the Iñupiat, who were shorter. Bruce was the representative of the Iñupiaq North Slope Borough mayor, whose headquarters lay hundreds of miles away. Bruce had power. He took up the next item on the agenda, the gist of which was to urge the corporation to make over to the "city" (the Ivakuk municipal government under the White state of Alaska, *not* the Native Corporation, and very much distinct from the IRA, the Native Government) the land on which the village clinic stood. "It will be very much easier to register the title to the land that way," he argued. He looked over toward Micky Hoffman. "Micky and I have come to an agreement about it," he said.

"A point of order," said Micky. "I didn't agree."

Norman Agansagga, the chairman, came to Micky's support. "*We* wish the land to go to the Native Government, to the IRA. Then the IRA will lease it to the city," he said. "*Lease* it," he emphasized. The whole room murmured agreement. Bruce was shaken.

It was instructive to see how these solid Iñupiat gentlemen, who called each other by their first names, gradually willed the burly and much taller White man into a hunched, trembly state. At the beginning Bruce had it all pat. He could help these people, who were in Chapter 11, after all. He put it to them that the bankruptcy judge would easily accept their assignment of the clinic site to the city but probably would not do so if the assignment went to the IRA. All knew that the city's affairs were taxable, as distinct from the moneys and land of the IRA, which came under the federal government and could claim tax-exempt status like that of the Indian reservation system under the federal Bureau of Indian Affairs. Municipal affairs, on the other hand, were under the financial control of other authorities, first under the borough and then under the White state of Alaska, which boasted one of the most conservative governments in the country. Furthermore, the people of Ivakuk could place no assemblyman on the borough council, because the population at the borough headquarters was eight times as large as theirs. Although the corporation's funds themselves might be taxable after 1991, the IRA was the land body; that is, it was the tribe itself. It would be impossible to tax that, for it had the rights of an Indian reserve.[1] Bruce apparently did not want Ivakuk to have any part in such a "backward" system. Its people really should join the modern age, his argument ran. Underneath what he said was a hidden threat that the judge would push the corporation's Chapter 11 status into full bankruptcy if they were not cooperative—tribal status or no. That was how the chicanery over the Alaska Native Claims Settlement Act (ANCSA) money had tied them up.

Very reasonably, Norman reemphasized that it would be best to assign the site to the IRA. And again Bruce repeated his warning. Micky leaned forward and said with his usual quietness, "Look what happened about the power house site. The borough tricked the corporation [it is possible that money was passed, or threats were used] to assign the power house site to the borough, so now that tract of land no longer belongs to Ivakuk. Outsiders from now on have the right to interfere at will with the power house, and that right lasts to perpetuity. They could shut it down or do whatever they want to do on that site." At this the members shifted in their seats. [In the case of the clinic the borough could and did control the dissemination of information about the people's health.]

Micky's eyes watched like a bird's after a worm. I gazed respectfully at him. The opinion of the room had jelled without a sign. Bruce was hand-tapping with a paper clip. When his hand was raised it trembled. That trembling was a thing he couldn't stop. His voice still came over full of bureaucratese, but it was wavering.

A vote was being taken. It was unanimous. Bruce was informed that the meeting supported the IRA assignment. So he had to accept it. Nonetheless, he had already shown himself able to twist any agreement, as with the trick he had tried on Micky about an "agreement" earlier.

Then they ever-so-politely dismissed Bruce from the room, with a warm "Thanks, Bruce."

Here I report the sequel. Bruce's method was persistence. During the next few years I saw several times how it was done, how he got his way for a time. He did it by continually giving "legal" advice in a multiplicity of meetings, in which he wore the members down. Bruce succeeded—in control by lease, though not by ownership—in this project of the clinic land assignment, in another issue concerning the school playground assignment, and in yet another, a road to the freshwater lagoon. All the land concerned was thus distrained from the Ivakuk people and was controlled by the borough, and so by the state of Alaska.

In the widely read book by Thomas Berger called *Village Journey: The Report of the Alaska Native Land Review Commission* (1985, 73–74), Paul Ongtooguk said this about Iñupiat land:

> I believe that if the vast majority of Alaska Natives were given the opportunity to either kill or die for their land, most of them would do just that if it was that simple. If you were supposed to shoot soldiers, or protect your land with firearms, there are more Natives than the Federal Government would like to think about that would be more than willing to do just that. It is not clear any more. Now when they are coming in after the land and they are coming in on these issues, they come not with soldiers but with people carrying briefcases. If you shoot somebody carrying a briefcase, then you are just a criminal, it is not an act of war. . . . There isn't any clear way for the people to protect their land. ∎

October 5, Monday. At this point I was back in spirit experience. That evening I dreamed I saw a man who was having to carry a whole pile of stuff like window glass—it had something to do with my house. Then I recovered consciousness. Then I dreamed again of some awful fault, some penalty I would have to pay. These were waking dreams, and I at once recorded them. [Later, on December 7 and November 10, I recorded how these two dream pictures occurred in reality (see chaps. 7 and 6).]

On the same day one of the older girls told me this: "My

brother Peter's seen the man in black who scares people at night. Very scary. He floats above the ground and has these black wings. The ones who saw it prayed out loud, real loud, *screaming* at it. It rose up in the air, then it became a black disk and disappeared. I tell you, if you have a cross and a picture of Jesus, it won't come near."

October 7, Wednesday. I was in the elementary school with the class of a young White teacher, writing family trees with the children. Several little boys accosted me and said, "Did you see the big animal last night? The Thing? It was scary."

"It was near those houses built on graves," said another. "About five in the morning. Peter Westfield saw it, Dionne's son."

"What was it? What was it?"

"A big black thing, very fat, seven feet high, large—"

"It had seven claws," broke in one boy, bouncing.

The teacher listened with fond horror. She was married to an Iñupiaq. "It's the full moon just now," she said. "They come out at the full moon."

"Wouldn't you be scared?" said a little boy looking up at me.

"Probably not. I had four elder brothers and had to fight them all. I had to grow up brave."

The teacher told me she had seen on the TV there had been a total eclipse of the moon at 2:00 A.M., but she hadn't stayed up to watch it.

I left the class at 11:20 and went to the post office. There I encountered Rafe Campesino, who lived next door to Dionne, and Daniel North, the Iñupiaq postmaster (who was also the magistrate). They were already in conversation about the night creature.

"You could see the footprints on the gravel—kind of footprints," Rafe was saying. Rafe was a Baptist Chicano from California and had lived in the village for some time. He played the guitar and liked health foods. He was a tall, good-looking man with black hair and a gentle voice.

"The marks were all in a row," he said. "There were holes in the gravel on each side, and there was a mark between them like a tail, like something dragging there."

"A tail?" said Daniel, the postmaster.

"Dionne and I compared times. It happened at 5:10 A.M. for both of us. It must have been the same creature. I never saw it, but I heard it. It sounded like a very drunk person."

"Human? It sounded human?" I asked.

"Yes, human. You could hear it. Words. Obscene words. I

couldn't repeat to you what. There was this sense of evil, and fear. A strong sense of evil." Rafe raised serious Mexican eyebrows. "Peter Westfield saw it. He was very scared."

When Rafe left, Daniel said to me, "Yes, those houses are built straight on the gravel, right on the graves. They should have been raised on posts like the others." He was accepting the account.

I left and went to the store. Clem was standing at the back looking at some hardware.

"Yes," he said. "They're all talking about it." His voice fell into the sing-song wondering tone of the spirit-experienced. "When you put houses over graves, the masters of the ancient science come up." ("What can you expect?" his tone of voice was saying.) "The masters are still there. The sha . . . ." He hesitated. I looked at him, wondering if he would say it. "The shamans. They were the masters."

"They weren't all bad," I said.

"They were like we are, some good, and some bad. Some had too much to drink. Some were *irritated* by other people." His eyes widened. Then his voice became gentle. "They're going to have to recreate the old science."

Ed Tukumavik, at the language class, had also heard the story and accepted it. I, too, began to accept it, thinking of Ernest Burch's article (1971) on giant beings. Rumor reported that the footprint was eighteen inches long. I set out across the gravel in Dionne's direction, soon finding myself accompanied by a bunch of children.

"You going to see Pokeman?" they asked. Nobody was at Dionne's, which was at the edge of the village, so the children led me around the house to the back, where there was nothing but tundra between the outer row of houses and the mountains of the southern cape, twelve miles away. Here the children met with a tall youth. This was Peter. He was actually only twelve. The children stood around in awe as he pointed to where some heavy sticks lay crosswise on the ground, protecting certain significant marks that could be seen beneath them. These were two long scratches on the ground, six feet in length and six feet apart.

"It's the Domino Snowman," said a small boy, meaning the Abominable Snowman. Other versions, besides "Pokeman," "hooked man," and "the man in black," were "Satan" and "Bigfoot," though "Caribou Man" was mostly used.

"They've messed up the footprints," said Peter. "Look, I'll show you. They were like this." And in another place he drew on the ground the outline of an eighteen-inch foot with two pads showing within the outline. He drew five claws in front and two behind. About ten children had now gathered, hopping about importantly and getting excited. I took some photographs of the marks, then a picture of all the children posing cheerfully. They enjoyed that.

As we started back the children said, "There's Dionne." A stout figure in a wolverine-hooded parka stood in the street, a stationary figure between the houses. I went up to her and explained my presence. It appeared she did not like to have the children fussing around. We sent them off and went to her house to talk. She unlocked her outer porch door, then unlocked her inner door. The house was clean right down to the vinyl floor. We sat on the couch. She proceeded to describe the night in the same way that Rafe did. I realized it was not the night that had just passed, but the night before.

"It was about 5:15 in the morning. I woke from this awful nightmare. I heard something. A voice kept saying—"

"In English?" I asked.

"Yes. It said, 'I want to smash the house down.' It used a lot of swear words, obscenities," she said in a low voice. "I've been trying to keep such words away from Peter."

Dionne rose and showed me how she lifted the window shade and looked out.

"Peter looked out and saw this black thing, thirty feet high. I screamed! I shouted at it, 'Go away! Go away in the name of Jesus! Jesus! Jesus!' Like that. The name of Jesus. And the thing backed off. It ran down that Honda ramp there and just disappeared."

As Dionne talked she was by no means in a jelly of fear. She explained, "A lot of friends have been in to sit with me right through the night. They said, 'Dionne, you have faith.'"

While telling me this, Dionne looked up at a picture on the wall that showed Jesus praying at Gethsemane, and also at another showing the Last Supper.

"See, my parents passed away. I'm lonely," she said. "My mother went three years after my father, because she missed him so much."

"I know how she felt," I said. "My husband, Vic, died four years ago. I felt lonely. I felt I hadn't got anyone to back me up any more. And I felt it was my fault he died. Well, I suppose it wasn't. But you need friends." We hugged each other with tears in our eyes. I couldn't help considering the house a good one. How could Dionne vacate her house, even though it was built on the graves? The spirit would have to get used to it.

I came home tired. I had made a great many visits that day back and forth on the loose gravel.

October 9, Friday. In the early hours of the night I was awakened by a huge CRUNCH on the gravel outside my window. It was an enormous noise, as if an elephant had landed from a height on one foot. I listened, a little excited, but could not work up any fear. What could it be out there? There was dead silence. There were no sounds of footsteps going away, no sounds of a Honda engine, no flutter of wings, just perfect silence. I raised the curtain. The window pane was covered with dewdrops, so that I couldn't see anything. I listened once more, but there was not a sound. So I went back to sleep.

In the morning Carrie said she too was awakened by the sound; moreover, she felt the house shake. She felt a strong sense of evil that she found very scary, also a feeling of cold. She had heard me move the curtain but had said nothing. I was pretty impressed by now. I got dressed and went outside and around to the back. I saw some very recently disturbed dirt in a sandy yellowish place near my window. The dirt was damp and stirred and looked as if it had been disturbed four or five hours before, not much more. I took out my notebook and quickly drew a picture of what I saw. Two long grooves joined in a fork showed in the dirt, about eighteen inches long and about three inches deep. I even fetched the camera and took a picture. I looked for some sign of a big single depression that might have been made by whatever caused the "crunch" sound. But there was nothing, only the scratch marks. A bird was the only thing I could think of, an enormous bird with one foot. But why was there no sound of flapping afterward? Was it a meteorite? Yet there was no sign of boiled slag, no large object that hadn't been there before, no big depression in the gravel. The sound had come from the surface, not like some underground movement of the permafrost. Was the thing partly material and partly spirit? I myself had felt no evil, just my usual sangfroid. Nonetheless, the facts faced me, the sound and the marks.

Rafe came and looked at the marks later, but said nothing.

I was pleased by the series of events. Here was an interesting conundrum, rich material. It filled me with wonder and excitement, much as it had the crowd of Iñupiat children. In a sense the children, in their love of knowledge and of anything strange, were more like anthropologists here. The events were an "object" to them. Nevertheless, when talking to Clem, I realized how serious this manifestation was. I could not be above the events, any more than I was above the church eucharist, or above the corporation meeting; I was certainly not above Caribou Man. I was embedded in Ivakuk: everything that happened there thrummed through me. I was riding along through the calendar with the people that year, in the same vehicle, as it were, and was subject to the same things they were.

With regard to Caribou Man, the whole village agreed he had indeed been in town. Anthropologists (Burch 1971; Sharp 1987) have recorded Native Americans' accounts of giant beings that include animals of various kinds, fish, and caribou-legged men. The figure of Netta's eagle (tingmiaqpak, literally "big bird") was one of these, the shamanic eagle who was said to have given culture to humankind. What the appearance of these animals implied, what it meant, I did not know. But just as the Iñupiat were doing, I wanted to learn what I could about such appearances, from their occurrence.

In this case the appearance of Caribou Man was the herald of a downward swing of morale in the village, in which I, too, was caught. Only minor ripples of the village troubles are included in this account, but serious ones had occurred, as they would in any small community. I could sense the flow of feeling in the village, the flow of gossip, the swirling currents that changed, grew, and sometimes exploded. And they were seasonal, at least in the year of my visit. This was social process rather than social anatomy. All societies appear to experience such flows. And in Ivakuk the flow also ran freely into what is termed a nonempirical dimension or level. When it did, the people concerned knew it and never failed to marvel. Carrie and I felt the same. The people were used to it—yet even so they were awed by the appearance of Caribou Man. ▪

October 11, Sunday. I had not even tasted whale meat yet, nor had I come into contact with the world of subsistence hunting. I hoped the contact would come soon, because I was impatient for the next stage.

5

The Taste of Sea Mammal
Awakens Iñupiat History

October 11, Sunday. Carrie and I were sitting at the Jacksons' table watching Margie bring out two ulu knives, which she proceeded to whet, one against the other. What was she going to do? Clem went off to his shed and returned with a platter and a full, heavy bag of something. The following poem tells what happened next:

Clem has a blood-red dish, a long wooden platter
    stained with red blood.
Clem took from the poke a heavy sagging slab.
        It filled the platter end to end.

        The meat showed strata.

        The surface was dark gray. This was walrus—
            its skin is impenetrable.

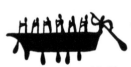

        We took the ulu knives, Margie and I:
            they're like halberd blades, short, with neat
            bone handles—
    it's like slicing with a half moon
    of tarnished steel. Clem
        had filed at the great curved edge and it shone.
We began to slice.
Margie's wrists looked slender. She turned the slab over
    and took the black-red meat first,
    slicing to the fat.
It swung open; she pressed surely
    and turned the blade as it passed.
Now it tore into the gristle, bounced and tore.
She persisted. And reached the coconut fat,
    cut it into crisp squares, then tackled the skin.
Yes, she cut the skin: the knife pressed nearer and
    nearer the wood, the dark gray parted at last—leaving
    the wood grooved.

I tried.
And I knew the mammal's regard for its skin by that last rending.
It was tough.

Margie put the meat on to boil; a rich pungent steam smelling somehow of fishy geraniums filled the room. That animal had eaten seafood, all right. Clams. The elder daughter made cornbread and chocolate cake; then Margie set out solitaire cards for herself, and we all talked. Clem said that if you send back the walrus's face into the water, the walrus waits for its relatives to come back on migration; then it takes on a new parka.

The unique odor hung around the kitchen. It released something in Clem. He stretched his arms out over the table and fingered the cards, then launched into a stream of narratives that seemed to hang together in a way of their own. He liked to talk, his flat, candid face upturned, his voice slow, and he did not like being interrupted. He told us that when he tried to talk about shamans at an elders' conference at the borough center they would not allow such items to be published because of the disapproval of the Christians.

First he showed us his big walrus hook for retrieving the walrus after it was shot. This was about six inches long and consisted of a large plug of bone set with two double two-and-a-half-inch hooks on either side, with a bobber for winter hunting and a sinker for summer. Attached was a strong nylon cord.

At this point Clem took out of his pocket a coil of leather ribbon about half an inch wide. He unwound it. Bound to the end was a large, dull red bead with knots at the top and bottom. He told us it was shamanic and that he wore it around his forehead when hunting. "Tulungugraq, the creator, wears a raven's beak set in the middle of his forehead," said Clem, and he began to tell us Iñupiat history. "The word *Iñupiat*," he said, "has been translated by Whites as 'real people'. This is fifth grade stuff. It means 'original inhabitants'. Okay?"

Clem flunked history at high school because he gave Iñupiat history in his assignments instead of the White history of Alaska.[1] His Iñupiat history went like this: "At first the world was quite flat. The raven god, Tulungugraq, took his kayak and went toward the east. He saw something under the water. He came up to it and thrust in his harpoon. He dragged, and he dragged, and he dragged, and up it came. It was the mountains. They rose up as you see them now.

"God, Tulungugraq—from *tulugaq*, raven," said Clem—scholar as he was—"created the world at Ivakuk, at a mound down at the end of the beach, where my grandmother Netta and my grandfather Kehuq used to dance. Most dances were rituals. For instance, the dance to the new moon in thanks for the walrus, whales, and so on that were not yet caught: that was a ritual." Clem said the Christians would not allow the moon dance.

"Yet it was a surprise and a pleasure for the Iñupiat to hear from the missionaries that Tulungugraq had a son. We *knew* about God already," he went on gently. "We knew about shamans traveling under the ice. My grandmother Netta's traveled—she's traveled many times before this illness. She's left her body, she's had out-of-the-body experiences. She's done that."

Then back to the history of the mountains. "When Tulungugraq created the world, there were mountains and land all the way to Siberia. Where there's ocean now, there used to be a freshwater lake. Geologists have found signs of it. Where the Diomede Islands are now, there used to be a river running between. Later the sea came in between Alaska and Siberia; and there'll be land in between again some time in the future. Now the U.S. military has DEW line points all up and down the coast, early warning stations against Russia." And Clem told us information about politics that I just didn't hear. It went in one ear and came out the other. I couldn't jump from ancient to modern history as he could.

Then he went on to the creation of day and night. [One version of this account, which I had heard elsewhere, started with a preliminary event. Tulungugraq wanted a certain woman. He could not get her, so he became a small seed, which she swallowed in her food, and she became pregnant with him. When he was born, he was a mischievous child and "broke his ball."] Clem took up his own version at this point: "Tulungugraq had three balls of light in his house, up high. One was very bright, one bright, and one not bright. His little daughter wanted a ball to play with, so Tulungugrak took down the middle ball with the pleasant light. He took it outside and ran with it, shouting 'Light! Dark! Light! Dark!' and 'Day! Night! Day! Night!' A man came up and struck him a blow. The ball exploded and nothing of it remained; but it was now 'Day,' and afterward 'Night' came, and day and night followed as we have them now. If the ball hadn't smashed, we'd have had eternal day."

Clem referred to another oral history. (The Iñupiat would prefer the term "protohistory," not "myth," for such accounts.) This was one that was well known and told in several versions. Now Clem said very briefly: "An early shaman married his sister here in

Ivakuk. It was incest, and they had to leave."

Netta took up the narrative. She called the incestuous couple "gods," not shamans. "The sun goddess and the moon god were sister and brother. The sun goddess used to sleep alone in her sod house, but one night in the darkness a man came into her house and lay with her. She couldn't see who it was. This happened again on many nights after that. At length she became inquisitive and found a piece of charcoal. That night she marked the man on his face with the charcoal. When the goddess went to the qalgi meeting house the following day, one of the men had charcoal on his face. It was her own brother. The sun goddess was so angry that she took a knife and slashed her breasts. The red blood poured out, and you can see the blood when the sun sets at night." Clem added that after the discovery the woman prepared food for the man to eat, and in it she put her own blood, feces, and urine.

Clem also described how the incestuous couple were banished for their deed. "The man went into the moon, and was cold. The woman went into the sun, and thus they were kept apart. You can see the light of the moon-man a little bit more each night while the new moon grows to the full. The man is gradually opening the door of the moon and letting the light show under the door. Around the time of the eclipse of the moon, when the couple finally get together, the man shaman travels in his spirit form for four days [the classic period for an Iñupiat shaman trance]. If he's away any longer he'll die and never come back. We therefore hope an eclipse won't last too long. Similarly, the sun-woman shaman travels for five days when there's an eclipse of the sun."

Netta showed me two bone masks made a long time ago by her husband, Kehuq, the old man who now continually shuffled about in the house. Both of the faces had upright ears on the tops of their heads like animals. The sun goddess was marked with vertical tattoo lines from mouth to chin, which were the woman's tattoos, while the mask of the moon god showed labret knobs below its mouth, one on each side—the man's traditional facial adornment. But the significant difference was in the human ears, the ones on the sides of the faces. "See," said Netta. "The sun goddess has large ears because she has sense. The moon god has no sense at all. He is stupid, and look at this, he has no ears. It is stupid to commit incest."

Clem continued with more history: "In the old days the Athapaskans invaded the Arctic. The Eskimos drove them out onto a promontory in Labrador and starved most of them to death. One Indian woman was left. She refused to marry an Eskimo, so the

Eskimos mated her with a dog. She gave birth to eight offspring, four human boys and four dogs. The boys grew up and they became very violent, like dogs. This history of the four boys is maybe the same as the one they tell down among the Hopi, who have a history of four sons who were red, white, yellow, and black. They became the founders of the four races."[2]

While Clem was talking, the walrus meat was cooked. The slab of meat now steamed in the middle of the table, which was well supplied with pilot bread, those hard and nourishing ship's crackers or hardtack, and mustard, and cups of coffee, and cake for afters. Using ulu knives, we cut the walrus into tiny long fingers, one-quarter inch by one-quarter inch thick, dipped them in mustard, then chewed hard. The meat was very good, a hearty, warm-blooded sea mammal taste. I had tasted it before. Where? Of course, in Stork margarine in England in World War II, when Clem was only a tiny child and Margie not yet born. Many whales died at that time for the manufacture of margarine. It was this taste, these sense impressions, that stirred up my early memories, even those of many days of fear when as pacifists in the war Vic and I had been ostracized, and even further back when as the difficult child of the family I was sent off at the age of eight to a boarding school situated in a village built on a gravel spit.

Here I was in the warmth of a family in a village on a gravel spit. The taste of walrus grew on me, I ate it and felt fine. I had been running a cold, but it was now improved, and my headache went away. Finally, Carrie and I left the adults watching an Agatha Christie story on the TV. When we walked from the house, the children "followed" us, that is, they came with us, and we were all very affectionate. On reaching our own house I taught the boys how to make origami paper toys until it was time for them to leave. At 11.45 P.M. we heard on our CB radio a gentle voice saying "Goodnight," followed by another tender "Goodnight," then another and another; then, greatly daring, I picked up the mike and said "Goodnight"; then several voices joined in. Then one said, "It's too early." At last one more said, "Goodnight, Ivakuk," sweetly; then another said, "Goodnight, Ivakuk." Carrie said to me, "Hear that? It's great." My eyes ran.

October 16, Friday. Down the school corridor I noticed Dick Kuper, my fourteen-year-old classmate in the Iñupiat class, with Ava, the sixteen-year-old daughter of the other leading Ivakuk healer, Suellen. Young Ava was also a healer herself. Her arm was affectionately slung around Dick's neck. Dick's superb shoulder muscles were showing under the sleeveless singlet he was wearing. Dick was going to be a father.

In the language class the students would suddenly connect with the language and toss out fine expressions one after the other, each with its clicked and clashed consonants, along with the undulatory vowel, then a short vowel trapped in the last "q" like a fish on the line—that "q" itself like the fishhook, constituting a deep back-throat closure after the wave of the diphthong: *tauqsigniavimuni-aqtuq* "He's going to the store." There was no doubt that their pronunciation was majestically sure, however much the language was said to be losing ground.

That night I noticed my Iñupiat parka lying at the foot of my bed with the wolverine ruff standing up like a living thing. It almost frightened me. The day before, Kaglik had seen me wearing it and said, "You're an Iñupiaq now." Kaglik kidded me a good deal.

October 21, Wednesday, 8 P.M. Several participants, myself among them, sat on the floor along the school corridor, facing the library entrance, with our backs to the gym wall. Clem and his drumming group had selected this place to practice for his troupe's performance at the upcoming Alaska Federation of Natives meeting in Anchorage. Kaglik was there, and Seth Lowe, and Joshua, a young man with black hair that was wild and long and a broad, loose smile, and many others of the Jackson and Lowe extended families. Even eleven-year-old girls in the group were performing very well. I watched the light way the men let the drums waft softly down upon their drumsticks for an initial muted stanza. The second stanza was in full volume. Seth's drum sounded deep and sonorous when he struck it harshly on the rim from below. The combination of harshness and plangency was peculiarly attractive. The rhythm itself consisted of a determined double strike, *"Du-dum, du-dum,"* along with an "ah-yah-yah" sound of vibrant singing, the tune of which rarely changed notes but suddenly ended on the note above the dominant, a strong note, and yet it rested unfinished as if off the ground.

Then the dancing began: first was old Tookruk with the lean face, in her parka patterned in long brown vertical lines, a spreading red fox ruff laid back on her shoulders. She was dancing and bending her knees with grace, never taking her feet off the ground. She too was a healer. Fat Seth danced, using footwork because he was a man, giving forth with a quick stomp with one leg while making sudden, vigorous gestures here and there—a nimble performer of seventy years old. His face was full of chubby wrinkles, and his black eyebrows projected vertically up and out one entire inch. He was all alive, a real Lowe.

I kept hearing the boom of the taut drum skin along with the slap on the rim. Clem was singing, and his voice had the same bite-plus-sonority as the drum sound, and so did the other voices. Most of these songs were Clem's. He owned 120 of them. Songs were usually owned by an individual, and they were shared at these times.

I found I could not help singing along and even imitating the hand motions of the dance as I sat and watched, because the rhythm absorbed me into it. In front of us all, blatantly staring at us on the school library wall, were posters of Boris Karloff as the Frankenstein monster, another of a skull with picture eyes and a picture nostril hole, and a Mr. Hyde monster man. Halloween was approaching. The Iñupiat drums played out their simple/sophisticated ancient music while I eyed the green face and scarlet mouth of Karloff.

Now Clem was dancing the great bird, the tingmiaqpak. He stomped and twitched, seeing nothing of what was before him, his strange, flat face in semitrance glaring this way and that, arms awry and then uplifted, down and away, then dizzily aloft, until the climax came and something seemed to spring upward from him, although his left foot was rooted to the ground. There was a clap of genius like thunder. The drums quit on the offbeat, and it was over. I never saw him dance so well as at that time. He told us afterward that he was needing food for his family, and dancing brings the caribou. "Dance," he said. "That's the way to do it." Indeed, many caribou did come that winter: we were eating caribou all the time.

Here Clem was working with his body, in actual performance, as well as verbally giving the young their traditions.

The same evening in his house he gave a further account of shamanism. "There is a man at the point with long ears and a big tail. He can hear everything we say. Once a shaman went under the water in his ball of fire in order to help a sick young man. He arrived at the animals' house under the water. The animals' parkas were hanging on the wall just like ours. These parkas were their fur and flesh. The animal/humans sat in this room and the man with the big ears was among them."

"The man with the big ears can hear us now," I thought. I looked at Clem sitting at the table, Carrie around the other side, and myself on this side, and thought, "He can hear us. This is yet another sign of the connectedness of all with all."

Clem went on, "Inside the animals' house the shaman saw the

sick young man lying down. The shaman asked a favor of the animal people, 'Let our relative come back and not die. We need him
to hunt for us; he's young.' So they let him go. At that moment,
back in the village the young man lying on his bed began to get
better, and he recovered." [I noted this later as the classic Native
American shamanic soul retrieval. My own trip down a tunnel when
I looked for Netta's polar bear spirit was somewhat different. In
that trip I tried to blow Netta's spirit back into her. I later learned
to address the animals properly and respectfully, though it took a
long time before I saw the sense of actually talking to them. The
threads between the components of the environment, both living
and geographic, could not easily be detected without a relationship
of respect.]

Clem sang many songs to help me to learn the singing. I tried to
achieve the plangent native "Ya! Ya! Ya-ya!" beat, my voice following his rather uncertainly. I did at least persist.

There came a day of drifting snow, which, though not covering everything, kept a constant change going over the
ground on which we walked. These changes were more no-
ticeable than those made by the wheel marks in summer,
which were mere wheel marks in the gravel. The difference was
snow sculpts *itself*. The gravel was originally brought to the village
site in trucks to cover the tundra as a foundation; it was not
sculpted by the sea in the way the shingle was sculpted at the edge
of the water. The construction vehicles continually made a worse
mess of the already dumped gravel. But now the wind itself had
material to work with—the snow—and used it to spin beautiful
shapes around some garbage box or disused electrical pylon—reminding me of Clem as sculptor, with the electric drill that his
mind guided, shaping a chunk of walrus ivory into a delicate finger
ring with a whale on it.

The life of strategy, of constant adaptation, of the satisfaction of
greed that had been induced by commercialism, set side by side
with person-to-person interactions producing personal excitements
and satisfactions, all clattered along together in Ivakuk; and under
the force of great feeling, or fear, or fits of generosity, or tender
humor, took shape in a sculpted form, in a kind of evanescent natural beauty—then it was gone again, trodden down, then swept up
once more quite differently into yet another shape. I continually
saw hints of the old culture, and I saw the joy taken in little children. For instance, I saw Atiq, six weeks old, resting on her father

Clem's knees, and his quiet voice above, both of them utterly satis-
fied for the time; wee Anna toddling out of the post office in front
of her mommy, Anna embodying the total love poured into her,
her round face full to the brim with that knowledge, like a
madonna.

All would get swept up and circulated again; one example was
the immediate reuse of the name of someone who has died, the
name going to the next sister or brother in the local version of reincarnation—implying that the spirit of the recently dead might come
into an already living person. The name equalled the spirit; that is,
in a kind of nonordinary time the name of a child "came" to a parent, and at the time it was bestowed, the reincarnated spirit was in
the child—it would simply be there. Another example of the circulation was bingo, immensely popular in Ivakuk, a game that poured
every loss and most of the gain out and back into the social body.
This principle of circulation happened to be basic to Ivakuk and
many other hunting societies. The population was nonstatic and
never stayed at home for long. People stood lining the inner walls
of the post office, waiting for mail from outside; they went hither
and thither on Hondas; they were forever changing jobs in a floating, casual way that I could not catch up with; or they were away at
the inland river in the fish camp, a camp that was temporary by def-
inition. The children grew up not structured, not in "good order"
in any way. They were all set to rise and overflow upon the older
generation: their activity came over in many Western eyes as
wicked, inconsiderate, and destructive. The children were out there
in the flux, unaware that flux was an Iñupiat trait, until they approached middle age, when the knowledge at last became conscious. But there was a band of golden, living consciousness that
never completely went away.

Later, in deep winter, I often saw a golden band at noon on the
southern horizon. This also described the shaman's golden safety
path in the storm. ∎

October 25, Sunday.   The Jackson parents were away with
the Ivakuk Traditional Dancers troupe, performing at the Alaska
Federation of Natives annual meetings. Their return was delayed by
further business. Carrie and I were babysitting their family this
evening until their arrival home. Marco, Clem's little boy of seven,
was the chief protagonist this evening. He was not Margie's son,
but Clem's by a previous marriage. He was one of Clem's children
who had inherited his great-great-great-grandfather Kehuq's

shamanic second sight. He was an absolutely solid little boy, built like a minitank—and in this he resembled Vic, my late husband. Marco was active, enormous fun to be with, button nosed, and had a brown face, dark pink cheeks, and brilliant eyes that looked straight at me with a secret grin under his serious thatch of hair. He would charge at me and hug me, whump.

Waiting for Clem to come home, I tried to keep the children amused with paper cutouts and other games. They got restive. Marco flung his arms around the table. "Where *is* he?" He meant his dad.

"He'll come."

Marco wailed incoherently. He lost his temper over something. He wailed again. Then he settled down to a prolonged *in extremis* crying that nothing could stop. It was a roar as in a four-day storm. I couldn't help finding it very satisfying, the abandon, the theatricality of it, his head nodding and rising, the total give-out under the tension of waiting and waiting for Dad to come back—so that all he could do was yell to the heavens. God, how I loved it. I turned around from my own old tired yell to the heavens about Vic's death to hear a tiny comrade yelling in my stead, with such physical strength that I gloried in it. Marco was a Hercules of yelling. And his tempers—they were absolutely without reason, a terrible statement of "To hell with it all." Maybe I was going to be sorry I said this, but I loved it. Marco knew I liked him; he was a conscious little boy and was actually fascinated by life.

On a previous occasion when his father was in Anchorage and Marco was at home in Ivakuk, the boy woke up in the night and screamed, "They're killing him with a gun!" It turned out later that at that precise moment Clem had been held up by a gunman in Anchorage. Fortunately, Clem was able to escape. When Clem heard what his son had said, he knew what kind of person the boy was. Clem knew that Marco could also "go into the future" as he put it, and he valued him. ∎

That night Carrie and I sat through Marco's hollering for a long time. Eventually the Jacksons did return safely, and everyone was happy.

October 31, Saturday. Something was up in Ivakuk on this day. Soon we discovered that a festival was in progress at the bingo hall, the festival of the Whale's Tail. Carrie and I peeped in at the porch of the Bingo Hall, where a crowd of young men in woolen caps was hanging about. As we peeped in, our noses immediately registered a high fishy, cheesy smell. People were pushing through, keen to get inside. Once in the hall, we saw that Dora Lowe Nashanik was in command, ulu knife in hand. She was her usual large, busy self, stationed in the middle of the floor, which was now covered with flattened cardboard boxes on which lay several two-foot-thick disks of hard, white whale fat, still covered with black skin. So this was whale meat, *muktuk*. Most of the fat was finely marbled with pink veins where the flavor was developing. These tail sections had been cut from the whale that Dora's husband, Robert, had caught the previous April. His whale was the one to be honored on this occasion because it represented the fifth whale catch in his lifetime. Dora, his wife, was therefore the principal meat divider and distributor. Robert's stocky figure was to be seen over on the other side of the hall in front of the oil stove. He looked modest and responsible, notably without emotion. Robert's money income for the expensive task of whaling came from his janitor's job at the school, a job he performed in an equally responsible manner. Robert was the brother of Timothy and Suellen, he was the uncle of Suellen's daughter Ava, and he was the nephew of Netta Jackson, all of them healers, as he was himself. Netta's Aunt Judy had been both healer and shaman.

At Dora's feet squatted a dozen women busily cutting up the slabs of meat with their ulus. The women were daughters, daughters-in-law, and nieces of both Dora and Robert. All these relationships had to be exploited in the huge task of whaling and cutting, and although there seemed to be a patrilineal tendency in the inheritance of whaling equipment, the bilateral character of the kinship system was opened before my eyes in this scene in the Bingo Hall.

The women cut off pieces of whale skin and fat, that is, slabs with about half an inch of black skin and an inch of fat. It was these slabs that were called muktuk. They threw the pieces into a number of zinc baths and steel bowls that were waiting ready. Dora skated about on the slippery, oily cardboard, dodging the whale vertebrae and exuberantly shouting instructions—the wild, tubby benefactor of all, handing slabs to people here, there, and everywhere, flicking them and almost throwing them in some cases, accompanied by a terrific squeal of laughter. She gave a little freestyle dance with her arms out, very pleased. And all the while Robert stood quietly on one side.

This was quite different from what I had imagined a whaling captain's wife to be like. From the books I pictured her as an obedient, modest, and quiet woman, not looking about her, a patient

Griselde in fact, probably thin, full of prayer for her seaborne husband and thus "drawing the whale." Not this huge jolly female.

Women gift recipients kept arraying more bowls on the side to await the progress of distribution. The remaining masses of meat in the middle consisted of clumps of sawn cylinders much as if a tree had been cut down and the trunk sawn into cylinders. You could see at the center of each piece the five-inch-thick spine bone and the gristle surrounding it.

I went and sat down with Netta, feeling jealous of the others who were eating, anxious that Dora shouldn't forget me, and hoping I might be able to taste my first muktuk. Netta was using her ulu to cut up tiny strips that looked like extra-thin domino pieces an inch and a half long—one of which she handed to me. Ah! I ate it, gratified. Again, it tasted like the Stork margarine that I had been forced to eat in World War Two, the taste of which I now remembered with pleasure—why, I do not know. Netta gave me a three-inch-wide slab to take home. So this was the revered food, the whale itself, presented in such a dainty slice. There was one sliver of gristle in the middle that I could not chew, so I hid it in my Kleenex. Now the young men who had been waiting outside, who turned out to be the heroes of the school basketball team, entered in a line and were given slabs of muktuk, which they received in plastic bags held open for the meat.

Paper towels were in constant use. The cardboard floor was so oily and slippery that I nearly fell over as I went to talk to Claire. Very quickly the festival ended, and everyone took her meat home.

Later we were to see the same meat distribution at a similar festival in March. Although the fact was never referred to, the principal festivals occurred at the quarters of the year: the fall, the winter solstice, the spring equinox, and midsummer: four festivals. There were other features of this apparently formless affair. This feast occurred when the ice was beginning to develop, so that it was known as the celebration of the coming of the freeze-up. Many people in the village had been saying, "Why doesn't the snow come? Can't wait. Don't like this weather," and so on. They wanted the snow. Some said they needed the snow because then they would be able to use their snowmobiles. Traveling by snowmobile over frozen ground and snow was in fact easier than traveling on Hondas over loose gravel, or over tundra tussocks and bogs in the rain. But there was something more about the ice. It was almost as if the ice were the rightful home of the people and it had deserted them from June to August. There was something further still about the Whale's Tail Feast that I was not grasping, something that had to do with human communication with the animals. ∎

November 4, Wednesday. Today, walking down to the beach over dead grasses, I could hear a high, tense squeak even through the thick folds of my hood and ruff. It was the ice on the sea. I saw loose ice out at sea with open water in front, while near to hand much solid ice had grown in from the shore. In order to see the shore ice I had to mount the sea bank. Here on the bank I stood on soft, dark brown sand dunes resembling in form, if not in color, the white sands of the outer banks of North Carolina, and fringed with grass heads corresponding to the sea oats there, but smaller. Here the grass heads shone with a clear, golden color against the brown beach; and above, the whole land was overarched by the enormous sky. Blue extended over a quarter of the sky to the north, while to the west beyond the point, clouds spread in a series of huge veils tinged with pink. Down over the dune on the shore itself the tide was out leaving dark brown sand. Where the high tide had last come up, it had left a polishing and contouring of frozen seawater on the beach—a sheet of ice that lay in a long floor thirty feet wide, all of it set solid in a maze of bas-relief, so that treading on it felt like treading on forbidden ground. Beneath my boots I could see multitudinous pebbles enswathed with ice, embedded in the sculpturing. Alongside the water itself extended a line of bastion ice, a Roman wall of it. Further on I was walking on block ice created by the continual building effect of the waves, a line where the sea's own lips at the small cliff edge kept clearing away what it created while still creating it, hollowing it, even making a little hollowed-out cliff four feet high.

I could scent the sea air. A flock of seabirds was riding on a long channel that was clear of ice. Right out toward the horizon lay flock ice, and by the shore rose the breakers themselves, whose fingers continually created ice. The channel in between constituted a strip of freedom brought into existence by the sea's own restless action, which permitted an ice-free zone just behind the backs of the breakers, a narrow area that had not yet had time to subside into the gentle ice-flecked rocking that could be seen as far as the horizon. Birds had found this strip; they were like people spotting their special area in this wild ecology.

Except for the narrow strip that was clear, all the sea was flowering into innumerable tiny ice floes tinted pink from the blue-pink sky. Even the horizon behind could be seen ribboned with the pink and white colors—these were the snows of the northern cape, those visionary cliffs. I turned and walked west toward the point itself, choosing my path on frozen shingle close to the ice cliffs. I came to a wide curve arching to the left, then to the end of the land. And there beyond the curve of the hook was a little pond of open water with black things playing in it. They were seals. They poked up their heads and shoulders and had a good look at me; then one would lie down forward with a swift glide, showing four feet of dark body, followed by the swirl of its movement. There were thirty or so of them, looking, dipping, busy with their feeding. They were small spotted seals, *natchit*.

6

The Seal and Its Organs

A Prophetic Seeing

November. Some time back the postmaster told me that we might find a better house to rent in Ivakuk than the one we were in. He knew that Joanna Sivuq, Claire's mother-in-law, had a house to let. Unfortunately, it had been left a long time unused, so that the furnace and the electricity were out of order. Still, these things could be fixed because there were experts of all kinds in this Iñupiat village.

I was due to make a visit to Bristol to meet two Soviet medical doctors who were interested in Native healing. As it happened, this visit coincided with our house move. Carrie had meantime been joined by her Indian fiancé, a Nootka from Washington State. The couple promised to fix things up in the new house in return for free rent. If I visited Bristol, I would be able to use Bristol's well-stocked store to buy requirements missing at the new house: forks, cooking pots, duct tape for sealing windows, and clean-up detergent, as well as a large order of groceries.

November 10, Tuesday. The visit to Bristol had a high point and an extremely low one. I hung around the visiting Soviet delegation, hoping to steal a little time with the doctors. I heard they had gone to the museum to see the Iñupiat diorama, specially opened for them in spite of its winter shutdown. I hurried down the snowbound street to the museum but found that the doctors had already left. Since at that date I had not yet seen the diorama myself, the caretaker allowed me to peer around.

Suddenly the Iñupiaq woman organizer of the Soviet visit turned up, furious that I had entered the museum without her permission. Why she was so angry I did not know. Was she pro-White, and did she hate my newspaper letter on behalf of the Iñupiat's rights to their land? Had she mistaken me for a certain researcher who had wronged her people? Was my writing scurrilous? Was I a fraud? Maybe I was, because at the time I had not been assigned a grant and was not with an agency. The woman refused to listen to any of my protestations of innocence. With terrifying venom she marched me through the door and out into the snow. I stood there, feeling more than the cold. I was appalled. What had I done? The effect fell on me like a personal wound. However, I had to make some move, so I decided to trudge back to the hospital, where the Soviet doctors were making the rounds.

I soon found myself in the prefabricated hospital complex and, walking down the long passage, to my surprise I met several Iñupiat I knew, and eventually I caught up with the two Russian doctors, Dr. Vladimir Davidenko and Dr. Nikitin. We exchanged warm greetings and decided to go for lunch at the hotel. As the conversation got under way, the English-speaking one, Dr. Davidenko, told me about a shamanistic seance and cure he had witnessed not long before in a village in Eastern Siberia, two hundred miles from Anadyr. Dr. Davidenko told me that the patient had been suffering from rheumatic fever and was extremely ill. The shaman instructed the relatives of the sick man (probably Koryaks) to build two large fires close to each other, and he placed the patient between them. Dr. Davidenko told me he was afraid the patient would be burned, and he nearly stopped the proceedings. But the shaman was determined. He sang and played his drum, and after a time the man was cured, quite cured, said Dr. Davidenko. This sounded like the real shamanism and more like the African curing rituals with which I was familiar.

Later, I realized that the strong power of Christianity in Alaska, felt in all decisions over jobs and the details of human life, had suppressed shamanism more thoroughly than the relatively inefficient Soviets had suppressed it. The Soviets were cruelly heavy-handed with their own Saami, Khanti, and many others, wherever their arm reached, but apparently it had not reached everywhere.

These two doctors, like all Soviet visiting scholars at the opening up of glasnost, greatly desired to work with American researchers. They were urging the formation of an international arctic studies institute in the far north of Alaska, an establishment with which they could interact. But as things turned out, the Russian-Alaskan collaboration became centered for practical convenience in Anchorage. ▪

Later, while doing my shopping in the big store, I again saw Dr. Davidenko and his colleague Dr. Nikitin. They were upstairs in the television department. I found Dr. Davidenko in the act of fingering the price tag on an enormous TV set, $969. Both men gazed at the set, their eyes covetous. I quietly withdrew and did my shopping, not forgetting to include a pair of snow boots for myself and the things on my list for the house. Everything seemed so ample in this store, whose finances were not affected by Chapter 11.

That night in Bristol the horror of the woman's curse in the museum returned to me. I hardly slept. I intended there and then to give up research and anthropology forever. But life went on.

Some time afterward I thought again of the woman organizer's words. They had come like a sorcerer's curse upon me—a blast of agony. Then I realized it was the very blast of agony I had suffered in my dream in the night of October 5—the dream about some guilt that I had taken upon myself and its penalty of mental pain. The memory began to take shape so clearly that I looked up the item in my journal. There it was, and it appears in the entry above for October 5. ▪

November 11, Wednesday.   I was glad to be finally in the airplane with my parcels and on the way back to Ivakuk, where I would be able to move into the new house, a better place in spite of its many problems. Ivakuk was looking like home. In the plane my companions were the head health aide whom I had seen coming out of Netta's house and the traditional healer Suellen, Netta's niece.

The weather was fine in Bristol, but as soon as we reached the southern cape, a demonic gale smote us. The sea below was frozen in long white and dark swales. We seemed to be far out suddenly, trying to beat back in, and all the while the tiny plane shook and trembled violently. The health aide's hand went out to hold onto the seat in front of her. You could see the knuckles tensed. Suellen sat serene. No hand appeared holding on. The boy behind me looked a little nervous. I said a prayer. We were now flying askew over the village—our good village—and continued over the ice lagoon and beyond it over the ice of the north shore, then around and back into the teeth of the wind—we were being swallowed like Jonah, somehow aiming for the long gut of the runway. The runway lights had been turned on, although it was only 1:00 P.M. We made a perfectly ordinary landing and came to a stop.

The pilot—it was our old friend Marvin, who had piloted Netta—laughed apologetically. "This flight was supposed to be canceled. Anyway, here we are." Suellen smiled to herself, and the rest of us giggled nervously.

Marvin taxied us to the road junction. There was no bus. Of course: it was Veteran's Day, November 11. Marvin did not switch off his engines, and we somehow hoped he never would. Ah, two pickup trucks appeared out of the din. But whose were they? What was I to do, with all those shopping parcels to tote back home?

"Don't want to get out, do yer?" said Marvin, opening up the door and letting in a fiendish draft. We clambered past the seats toward the door and unwillingly negotiated the steps down to the ground, trying to keep our feet. My wolverine ruff was not tied up under my nose, so the wind blew straight at the trigeminal nerve centered on the left side of my nose—my weak spot.

I dimly saw the airline agent. It was Elana Lowe, the woman in charge of the store. She indicated a pickup. I lumped my things somehow onto the back, then hesitated to get into the cab—was this the right one? The result was that I lost my grip of the door handle, and the wind took me away.

"Help!" I yelled, and a man grabbed my hand. I struggled in and banged the door. The window would not roll up, but no matter; we made it home.

All night long in Ivakuk it was foul weather and very cold, with driving snow. That night Margie Jackson won $1,000 at bingo. As for me, I went to bed with a headache and took two aspirins.

Looking at this episode after an interval, I asked myself, "Why was Suellen so serene?" And an anecdote of Claire's came to mind.

Claire was on a plane trip with her relatives; the weather was tricky. As they started for the borough center, she saw a bright sharp line right across the sky—golden, not cloud-colored. The weather was bad, with sixty-mile-per-hour winds and cross gusts, very dangerous for flying. "But we flew perfectly steady all the way and landed fine." Claire related this in a tone of frankness and wonder, a proposition for our belief, a marvel that does happen.

These modern examples had an older counterpart. A shaman could alter the weather, Clem told us. Netta related that long ago she and her relatives had once been marooned by bad weather in their cabin upriver, far from home and without any food. The snow was falling so thickly that there was a whiteout; that is, no one could see anything in front of their faces. Her uncle Runiq harnessed the dogs to his sled and said, "Let's try to make it home." When the family loaded themselves onto the other sled, they could see nothing at all in front of them, just whiteness. The only thing to do was to follow Uncle Runiq. Suddenly before them the atmosphere opened up like a tube along which the air was quite clear. And there at the far end they could see Ivakuk and home. They simply followed Uncle Runiq's sled in the tube and came safely to Ivakuk. (The wonders of this man "Uncle Runiq" were told many times in conversations with Netta.) Annie Kasugaq had had a similar experience.

All I know is that Suellen was relaxed on our plane journey of November 11, and everything went well. My records of spirit experiences in Ivakuk included other triplets like these, consisting of my own experience, second-hand contemporary accounts, and accounts of events in more distant days. ∎

The Seal and the Prophecy

November 18, Wednesday.   Clem Jackson caught a four-foot ringed seal, a *natchiq*. As I approached Clem's house that evening, I could see it lying on the sled behind his snowmobile. Clem and his son lifted it into the house and laid it on some cardboard that Margie was rapidly spreading on the living room floor. Clem told me that Margie had put some fresh water in its mouth as a respectful act, "just as I offer coffee to you when you come. We give fresh water to sea animals and oil to land animals."

"A caribou can get plenty of fresh water up river; it's used to that," Clem continued. "We give it oil. In the old days the people drank oil, and dipped their meat in water, just as they dip their meat in oil now. In those days the world was upside down."

Later, I looked more into the matter of reversals. The reversals that Clem was teaching us here were part of the Iñupiat history of the world. Far back in time Tulungugraq, the Raven, had turned the world upside down, to the way we see it now. This was reversal as difference itself, that is, difference itself as the marker of the difference in the eras. The Iñupiat account of the reversal shows that there was once an obverse to the mortal world as we know it. Only after the reversal did we become conscious of what it was like before the reversal—we know it by default. Barbara Myerhoff in an important essay on reversals (1978) describes the ritual reversals enacted by the Huichol Indians of Mexico when they entered the sacred territory on their pilgrimage journey to gather peyote. They would say "Good morning" when they meant "Good evening," would say the sun was shining when it was the moon, and used many humorous verbal reversals, such as "penis" for "nose," once they were within the sacred land. Ritual reversals "reestablish the primordial condition of humanity, in other words, they banish time," said Myerhoff (1978, 231). Again, "Reversals accomplish many purposes and contain a major paradox. They emphasize the difference between [the ancient condition] and the mundane life, and the differentiated nature of the human condition" (1978, 235). In the world before Tulungugraq's act of reversal, people walked on their hands, as one version of the book of Genesis tells us the dead do, those inhabitants of Paradise (Graves and Patai 1966, 73). The very act of bringing in a dead seal switches a person back to that sacred time, and so the Iñupiat give it fresh water, the opposite of its element in the mundane world. This is clear from what Clem said. More than this, reversal "makes for a concretization and amplification of the ineffable" as Myerhoff put it (1978, 231–32). The seal lamps in the primordial Iñupiat days burned upside down—concrete enough. As for the ineffable, we cannot speak of it, but "inversion" itself is an extreme, amplified form of that ineffable thing, which is "oppositeness" itself, that which is "different," to use the healers' word—and very difficult to express. So we now appreciate how the big inversion, as big as could be—a somersault from our point of view—was the norm for humans and all things back then. What the present volume shows is that the Iñupiat reexperience it now, from time to time, as if back in the old era. They—and I—dream beforehand of what is going to happen, "banishing time," in effect. Uncle Runiq's deeds represent another instance. The philosophy of reversals encompasses more than our present philosophies. Native philosophies often do. ∎

The seal lay on the floor. I stroked the ring markings on the seal's fur, each ring about two inches wide, white on dream gray, stippled all over the wide, slack body. At the lower end stretched the big webbed feet-flippers, which I drew out straight in order to look at them. The web skin was strong and sensitive, black. A neat triangular tail appeared between the feet, adorned with a triangular ring mark to match the rest. The face was bloodied up and gashed in; the face was a good place to aim at because then the skin could be used whole, and moreover, the beast did not suffer so much. Clem had used a heavy shell. The sensitive nose was still there, with the whiskers spreading five inches long in bunches on either side. I drew the whiskers out. They were like a cat's, curving and sensitive. Like a cat's they must have sensed sonar. Then I spread the hands, short hands with five equal claws, and very beautiful.

"What do you use the skin for?"

"The uppers of mukluk boots. Sealskin pants. Jackets."

"How much does this seal weigh?"

"Ah," said Clem. "What do you think?"

I put my hands around the round body, straddled over it, and tried to lift it. I couldn't. I said, "100 pounds? 200? I'm thinking of sacks of corn. I used to be able to carry 100 pounds."

Margie said, "I'm 140 pounds."

"May I lift you?" I said, and she let me try. I could, just a little.

"There you are," I said. "The seal is heavier."

While the seal lay on the floor, we ate caribou soup from a huge stew pan standing in the middle of the table. Pancakes and pilot crackers lay at hand, also plenty of whale muktuk, the delicate skin-and-fat slivers that tasted so good. Clem put Netta and me at the end of the table. "Two great ladies," he said. We grinned at each other, she with her wrinkles and her eyebrows raised in light and fun, I in sheer enjoyment. Now that she had recovered, she was going to begin her dancing instruction again in the school. She was seventy-eight and certainly had enough energy for the job.

The food reminded me of English food in the late twenties. This food had actual substance: this was food! Not an invented version of food, as in the present-day stores. It is as if the food producers nowadays make something to look like meat, look like fat, look like fish, just as laminated plastic can look like wood. What we were eating in Ivakuk was actual, real food after all those years, food for the body and soul. So I felt surprisingly good when I ate it, and felt I would live forever.

November 18, Wednesday.   Margie came through on the CB and told me they were going to skin the seal at 1:00 P.M. This would include all the processing.

"I'll give the language class a miss and come," I said into the mike. She laughed.

When I arrived, there was quite a crowd in the room. A young

Jackson woman was there to learn seal skinning, along with Margie, who was practicing it. Lena, an older one, was there to teach. Also present were Edwina, two Jackson hunters, the local Jackson basketball star, another young woman with a new Jackson baby, and the teenage daughter. All were siblings or cousins or children of Clem's, and everybody present was likely to receive some of the meat.

People went back and forth sharpening ulus. Margie, with the aid of the others, managed to turn the seal over. I watched.

She took the knife and made the first cut into the seal's parka, into its fleshly envelope, first making a shallow cut into the fat, right down the belly from the neck to the tail, then a cut across the neck making a T. There was deep, white fat inside. I thought, "How does the seal turn its fish diet into that intensely energy-laden fatty overcoat?" The digestive process must be nearly 100 percent efficient—turning protein into energy, first breaking down amino acids, which itself requires energy to achieve, then transforming those building materials into lipids (fats).

The cut that ran down the body of the seal was already wet with its own runny oil. Margie started on the fine skin, cutting inside it and gradually alongside it, tugging it off like a garment. She took a long time, going painstakingly around the legs and hands without slashing them off. She saved the claws for a necklace and the skin itself for the uppers of mukluk boots. The floor began to get slippery with oil.

Clem was in the back room with the baby, where I joined him. He sure did not mind that I had missed language class. We talked about that class, which was for ninth graders and higher.

He said, "How do they teach Iñupiat? They teach words—which are parts of words and mean nothing by themselves"—which I saw was true. We had been learning lists of words, usually a verb root, ending in the air, as it were, with a hyphen. Clem eyed me. "They've set out the way to learn it using the English way of speaking. The children are made to learn *English* Eskimo."

We went around to the kitchen, where Clem filled the electric water heater for tea. "Like 'running' in Eskimo," he went on. "Eskimos have all sorts of ways of running, fast, slow, down to the ice, for a long time, hunting animals." I was thinking too of "wanting to run, being able to run, going to run," all those internally inserted "postbases" in my grammar book—a multitude of adverbs and conditioning syllables that produced long words, each immediately meaningful as a whole, each one loaded with goodies like a seal's stomach.

Clem said to me, "You don't speak because you learn 'words.'"

You can't learn what to say just by knowing one word, then adding one other word, and then another word." He gave an Iñupiat phrase. *"Aqpanniangitchuq"* "He will not run." I couldn't say it. "You learn by saying things."

[I could see that the style of thinking implicit in the Iñupiat language was indeed quite different from the thinking implicit in English; Iñupiat had the same rolling connectedness as the Ivakuk "string genealogies"—those strings of kinship connections, relationships of siblings, half siblings, cousins, siblings-in-law, adoptive siblings, other children of divorced parents, even a pseudokin relation called *umma,* a person who is your namesake's sweetheart and whom you could kiss—all these strings that threaded through the village and around again, not in power pyramids of lineages but in horizontal strings, on a here-and-now level. I had come across "string genealogies" in the kinship system while writing down the children's family trees.]

"The children don't learn anything at all at the bilingual class—how can they?" Clem looked around in wonder, showing his gappy teeth.

"You're right."

He said, "I gave them the school curriculum at the borough, at the elders' conference. I wrote the curriculum they asked for. That was twelve years ago last year. Nothing has happened."

"What was in your curriculum?" I asked.

"Subsistence, sewing, history"—[note that he had been flunked in high school for substituting his own people's history for what the high school students were taught by college-trained teachers (see chap. 5)]. "Language, subsistence, sewing, history. Healing, dancing," he went on. "They should go side by side with the White subjects and should be *required.* Now, because the bilingual course is elective, they don't elect to take it."

I could see a school run with an Iñupiat curriculum. "A curriculum centered on Ivakuk," I pondered. "Climate, animals, hunting. The Whites have got education wrong." I looked at Clem's flat face turning toward me, his puzzled eyes.

He went on to speak of his efforts for political rights. "I told them about the bills in Congress that affected us, what each one meant. When I go to a meeting they know I won't say 'Yes' all the time; they'll get the truth. And they don't listen. All the last generation are yes-men." His voice went fluty, a little bitter. "They say nicely to the Whites, 'Is my tie straight? Do I look all right, sir?' They were taught to *obey.*" Clem's voice grew soft again. His eyes looked sorrowful. His mouth pouted, his lips apart. I became hot. "I'm not angry any more," he said. "I've done all I could. They don't listen to me now." Clem gave a parody of the anthropologist inventing meanings. "The anthropologists come up with ideas in their own heads about the way the system works. There's this anthropologist; he comes rushing in.

"'I've discovered the meaning of the *unipkaaq,* the old story,' says the anthropologist. 'A man takes a pebble into his house, one every day, and eventually the house is full to the top with pebbles. Then he takes one out every day. This is the meaning of the *unipkaaq.* What do you think of that?'"

"'It's not true,'" Clem answered the imaginary anthropologist, shaking his flat mask of a face in his slow way, his hair flopping. "It's very sad," he commented. [What was I to say? Too often the interpretations of the anthropologists bore no relationship to what the people themselves would say about their culture.]

"The early history *is history,*" explained Clem. It was a statement of fact.

Meanwhile, in the living room Margie had finished skinning the seal, so I took an ulu and helped her take off the blubber. The blubber was three inches thick, delicate and soft and comfortable. "When we cut the head off, the spirit can go out, and it'll grow another parka," said Clem. Its body would circulate in its eaters, its spirit would be separated and go to do its work of reincarnation, and the cycle would continue on its way.

"Look at the teeth," said Carrie. "Just made for catching fish." The teeth looked like dogs' teeth, but the canines were only slightly larger than the other teeth, unlike dogs' canines. They were small, neat teeth, healthy looking.

While I was cutting off the fat, once or twice I cut as far as the meat, which wasn't a good idea. I retained a thicker layer of fat after that. I had to press the ulu hard when circling around the tough sinews of the penis. At last all the blubber was off.

Now Margie bent over the seal and passed her ulu in a long line downward, opening up the chest and belly cavity. The great array of organs sprang into view, very dark red, almost black, glistening. I could see the huge liver lobes, at which I gazed, mesmerized. Dark red. Then an intricate maze of small intestines twelve inches across, dark brick in color. Then the broad, hearty tubing of the large intestine ridged like a vacuum cleaner tube. But all of it was delicate, set glistening and wet in the body cavity, packed neatly and efficiently and comfortably. I looked and looked. Margie drew out the liver. It was huge. She detached some of it, sought the gall bladder, found it, removed it—it was two inches long—and shoved the bitter little object into the trash can with the palm of her hand. She rejected the large intestine and took possession of the masses of small intestines. "We'll braid them," she said.

Braid them? In England they used to eat pork chitterlings fried—much the same body part. But not *braided*.

The round, notched heart, black: she took that. She threw out a knobby object, also the internally located testicles. At the sight I grew poetic, and thought: "Joyous beast, clothed in warmth, a swimmer provided with its own tropics, gamboling, shaped perfectly to live and grow fat in the freezing sea." And its sexual power . . . The penis, half an inch across, had just been visible before skinning at the exit of the posterior hole; the hole was an inch across. The penis was a small organ but no doubt a treasure to the beast.

Then the lungs, which reminded me it was an air-breathing animal. Margie threw those out. She now had everything ready for her teacher, Lena, to take over. Lena first saw to the meat division. She divided the rib cage neatly at the places where the ribs were naturally jointed, on the sides. Margie cut off the hands after Netta had shown her where to find the joints of the flippers. The joints were far back in the body, near the backbone—these were ball and socket joints. The dividing of the joints had to be done by old Netta herself. Netta knew where they were by feeling for them first, just as she felt with her hands when healing. She made the necessary cuts; then we saw the pale hollow of the socket and the small, pale sphere of the ball—the engineering of Nature herself.

Lena took over again. She divided the shoulders, then the belly meat, which she cut into four sections, then the backbone with meat on it, which she divided into two-vertebra sections. Netta had to show Lena how to get in between the vertebrae. The two of them dealt with the small of the back, which was very meaty. The body was now nearly cut up. To separate the ribs from what they called the breastplate, that is, the sternum, Netta pointed with her ulu along the groove in the breastplate from which the ribs sprang, showing the women that it was easy to cut there. The neck was very obstinate, but at last the head was off. It was all done.

Then it was a matter of plastic bags for the distribution. Because Margie was from outside, the meat went to the children of her and Clem, to Clem's relatives, to his siblings and half siblings, to his nephew the basketball player, and to his cousin, Wally, on Netta's side. Some went to Margie's sister, who lived in town. When Annie and I cut up seals later, the meat went to her and her husband, to her grown-up sons, and to a cousin on her side of the family who had helped hunt the seal—none to other relatives on her husband's side, though her husband would give some of his own share to his sister, old Joanna. So the balance leans where obligation resides, and this could exist on either side of the family. Annie, a local, was smart at recruiting crews from her side of the family.

The intestines lay in a bowl, and the pieces of blubber sat in two large bowls to allow the oil to drain out for the valued seal oil. Now for the braiding. Before this began, Netta taught Lena how to clean the small intestines. They were maybe twenty feet long. She did it by squeezing them all the way down to get rid of some of the half-digested material inside. Yellow-brown liquid poured out of the far end. I did some of this job, rather messily.

Then Lena cut a two-foot-long strip of the seal's blubber about an inch thick. She took this rope of fat and the top end of the long intestine in her hand, and wove the intestine around her index finger and thumb, keeping the rope of fat protruding from within her hand. Then she wove a new loop of intestine over the pointing finger and "cast off" the old one as in knitting; then she wove the intestine "yarn" this time under the rope of blubber, shifting around a bit, then around the finger next to the old loop and cast that one off; then she continued on similarly, all the time enclosing the blubber within a weird, knitted cable that began to emerge under her hands and grow long, eventually over a foot long. The finished cable was quite fat, three or four inches across. It looked beautiful, with regular plump loops, forming a cable with a square cross-section patterned all the way along. The rope of fat remained nested inside the finished product.

Everyone was proud.

"Now we'll boil it," said Lena. "It tastes good." Like sausages, probably, I thought.

I wiped up the worst of the blood, we threw out the oil-soaked cardboard that covered the floor, Margie mopped the floor, and that was that. The young women had been watching intently.

Here, then, were teachers of teachers, a true university. Netta was the emeritus, Lena was the professor, Margie the graduate, and I and those such as the teenagers were lowly freshmen. That is what I might think—a comparison that accorded with my own experience. But still it was one prototype of what education really is. Everyone was absorbed and perfectly happy.

November 20, Friday.   Annie Kasugaq, my neighbor, and I were becoming great friends. She would stump up my porch steps, enter at my shouted "Come in!" and flop into a big armchair, her snub nose cheerful and her hair in bubble curls. She was an overweight woman, a grandmother of twelve with more grandchildren arriving, and wife of a whaling captain. She spoke musically and not always according to English grammar rules [a matter I ignore in this book].

"One day we were down on the ice watching for whales. It was my birthday. I was looking out to sea and found my arm straight out, pointing, and I was shouting, 'There! There!' It was a whale, right near the camp. They caught it. They launched the harpooner in the boat by himself, and he put in the point. Then the others followed for the finishing of it."

"What a birthday present!"

We had a long talk about family. She was a Christian and often prayed.

"I've a headache," she said now. She pointed to the middle of her forehead.

I went over and felt it. The skin was alive with a twinkling sensation. "Poor Annie." I put my hand on the back of her neck. It seemed to me there was an easy unlocking of the pain and a giving of it away to me. I felt this from her. It was a faint perception, though. Annie sighed and said, "Thank you." I went to wash my hands.

November 24, Tuesday.   I went over to see Jim Agnasagga. Jim was another old believer, although he was a youngish man. He told me there were several good practitioners of the old arts in the village. Clem. Micky. Harold. Simon. Robert Nashanik. [I already had some idea of the kind about those people. Robert was a healer. Clem's dancing brought the caribou. Harold was a curiously gifted way finder. Simon knew about the now-dead elder Temek, who, he said, was the one that had gotten rid of the world's worst tyrant, Stalin, at a distance. And Micky, in the corporation office, was somehow—certainly not by monetary means—pulling the village out of bankruptcy. I could include Netta, but that is an account for later. And of course there were the principal healers, Claire and Suellen. On another occasion Jim described his own shamanism, very modestly. Quite a number of people. So was shamanism dead on the North Slope? Furthermore, what actually was going on in the drumming practices for borough competitions?]

After Jim Agnasagga had told me these names, I confessed to

him, "The fact is I'm studying healing here because I've seen some strange ritual healing in Africa."

"You'll need a whole year to study it here," he said.

"The healers used to be shamans, didn't they? The shamans weren't all bad?"

"You'd better know, there were two kinds of shaman, the good and the bad. When they tried to abolish shamanism, they got rid of the bad shamans, and the good ones turned into the healers. The healers use spirits."

"Animal spirits? A seal?"

"M-m. Perhaps."

"I'll tell you about what I saw in Africa. A spirit form," I said. "A big drumming ritual was going on. They were trying to get a bad spirit out of a sick woman by means of cupping horns. After a lot of trying—it was at the very height of the ritual, when everyone was drumming and singing like mad, and I was singing and clapping too—then, listen to this, the tribal doctor bent over the woman and out came this blob, big, that big." I showed a six-inch ball with my hands. "Gray. A kind of shadow. And afterward she was well."

Jim was listening carefully. I told him how Vic, my husband, had once brought a man back from the dead. "The man had a heart attack and his heart stopped. The medical doctor announced the pulse had gone. Vic put his hand on the man's chest and the pulse started again. Vic took his hand away and it stopped again. You can bet Vic put his hand back on quick and kept it there until the man recovered properly. The man was quite all right afterward. This happened in Chicago in about 1974. Yes, and I talked to the Soviet doctor Vladimir Davidenko, who actually saw a shaman cure a hopelessly ill man near Anadyr. I know those things."

Jim's eyes lit up at the stories. The man knew what I was talking about. He loved it. These days it was such a relief for me to home in on what I was really looking for in Ivakuk, to talk about it, and to find such a happy, relieved response.

In these conversations Jim often spoke in a kind of exploring voice, in spontaneous bursts, and so did I. He said, "The sick person has to . . . has to let the hands of the healer take away the pain . . . and the bad spirit, and has to hand them over." Yes. Jim and I *knew* this. And Suellen and Claire did.

I began to say, "It's what I felt inside Annie's head the other day when she had a headache—I felt her letting—" I couldn't put it into words.

"I know what you mean, I *know!*" he broke in. I leaned back, delighted. I knew he did. He was a young Victor Turner, age thirty-six. I was overcome.

He was in a construction job as a carpenter and a mechanic.

"It's a job," he said with his self-deprecating smile. He held out his hands. "I work with my hands."

We chatted on. "I'd like to see what you write," he said. "What do you believe in?"

"All the religions. Far more than the Christian religion. African spirits. Korean shamanism. South American shamanism. Japanese Buddhist redemption. Christianity, of course. And now the Iñupiat's religion." [I could have mentioned Judaism, Islam, Hinduism, the North American Indians' religion. There were so many.]

He positively wanted me to learn from those Iñupiat who were gifted. "Tell people here your story of the African healing," he said. "Whoever it is will come . . . you know . . . you'll—"

Late that night I felt my cheeks alive and burning warm from the cold. I had not felt my cheeks since I used to work on a farm in 1942. I was wondering how I'd ever be able to leave this place.

Then I suddenly understood the meaning of a curious experience I had had on July 19, 1987, before coming to Alaska.

That July in Virginia I participated in an experimental shaman session. We lay on the floor with our eyes closed while somebody beat a drum steadily. We were seeing whether we could go to the "upper world," that is, visualize some tree, mountain, ladder, or tall building, ascend it, then let whatever was out there take over.

The drum sound went before me. I visualized the ancient pile of Salisbury Cathedral. I entered the building with its curious, inverted arches, then climbed the spiral staircases to where the spire began. There was a rope extending from the ramparts to . . . before I knew it I was out on a fluffy cloud facing a monk in a long robe. I was not dreaming; these things just happened.

"What the dickens?" I said. This was all very corny. Churches, clouds, monks?

"Be quiet," rapped the monk. "It's not for you to criticize. Do as you're told."

I was somewhat impressed. My "visualization" was reprimanding me—or was it a visualization?

"Go on up a bit further," he instructed. There was another floor about three or four feet up. On this level I saw a whole bank of appliances along a wall. The wall was filled with CD players, stereos, VCRs, dials, and an enormous TV screen in which I saw something dark, very dark red—a sideways image of some internal organs, I thought, peering at it. Unusually dark red ones. They were internal organs all right, but they did not look ordinary, not like human organs. Elongated. Fatter. I was quite puzzled, but the drumbeat changed, and I was supposed to come back. Politely thanking the monk, I returned, opened my eyes, and told the others what had happened. No one could make anything of it. ■

I now understood that what I had seen in the TV screen was just what I saw when Margie opened up the innards of the seal on November 18. Now why should I have foreseen that event? Remembering the shaman experiment as I lay on my bed in Ivakuk on November 24, I put my hand down toward the bed frame to assure myself that this was real. My hand contacted my heating pad, so it must be okay. I was kind of upset. Tears came out somewhere inside me, seeming to soak, as it were, the subsoil of my head, my deepest consciousness.

Now in my bed my ears were picking up an irrelevant sound. The CB started to communicate, and Iñupiat voices came on in their sing-song game of "Goodni-ight!" alternating between kids and grownups. It must be the birthday party of Dora's grandchild. . . .

I felt nursed by the zero wind outside, by the CB with its quiet voices. I felt the puffy down sleeping bag over my tingling shins . . . childish voices. . . .

"Jesus," I said to myself. "They've got the quick, gavotte movement of a Beethoven symphony on the CB! It breaks my heart. I think the Choral, the most magnificent. See what I mean? . . . Such luck is evanescent . . . like the northern lights . . . anything permanent would be all the more mortal."

November 25, Wednesday. Jim's advice was soon to pay off. Claire came to my house and asked me pointblank what I was doing in Ivakuk. This time I did not have to say, "To write a scholarly paper on healing customs," or some such. I told her: to experience healing and spirit perception. That. I told her that in Africa I was at a healing ritual, helping, and at the climax of the drumming I saw a spirit body emerge from the back of the sick woman. And I told her again about Vic bringing back the heartbeat to the man who had died. That being so, how could I help believing in her work? What else could be my aim here?

Claire considered a minute. Then she said, "I'm tired. I have that pain in my rib. It happened when I had a Honda accident. It got my rib here. It's still bothering me after four months."

I was checking the oven and turned. "Shall I rub it for you?"

She didn't say yes but went to sit down at the table. She put her hand to a back rib on the right. "It's not badly hurt, but—but—" I put my hand there and followed where her hands showed the spot. Had she broken a rib? I remembered how in 1941 a horse had crunched my body between his cart and a gate, and how the pain had gone on for months. Maybe that had been a broken rib. Yes, there on Claire's rib was a clenched thing, about one and a quarter inches across.

"That's it," she said.

"Yes," and I showed her the size with my finger and thumb. "It's clenched up."

I merely caressed it, as Claire would have done. Around, and on top. The thing seemed to dwell greedily on that rib, scaring the body into believing it was sick. A lump, all right. It was body stuff acting up hard in the wrong place. I sighed. My hands knew this thing was sore. Now, astonishingly, Claire was letting the thing go into my hands. She let it go and let it go. The clenched part was mainly softish now, but I could feel within it a little long section still hard, say half an inch long. And I handled it a bit in the place where it was hard, inside. You get a little picture of it inside there. Now there was only the shadow left.

"That's better," said Claire, so I went to wash my hands. She told me later that the pain had not recurred.

I wasn't doing it. It happened from . . . doing the right action? Not exactly. From some . . . some "X" intervening when the two elements are there, that is, the person in pain, and a person evidently able to transmit it away.

The perception of the trouble did not appear to be extrasensory perception, outside the senses, but an actual fine sense—existing contrary to expectations—in the fingers, somehow resulting in the transfer of the ailment. This sense perception of the fingers seemed actually to exist; and there was a knowledge, a certain awareness in the human consciousness of a link between oneself and the sufferer, empowered by a kind of rushing of one's own consciousness into that of the other. This, whatever it is, is the concrete meaning of "sym-pathy," "feeling-with"; and it follows a palpable path, through the fingers' understanding. In this experience, it had something to do with the cast of feelings. When the feelings are open (they cannot be forced), the channels to the other person are open. Somehow nothing happens if the person is not sick; it is the hands' sympathy with the person's sick tissues that opens the way. The "sympathy" that passes is not only "energy" and heat; it is too personal for that. Whatever it is, it is the cause of the "opening" that takes place at the hands' contact with the sickness. That rushing of one's consciousness into the other person—that sigh—I think is exactly the spirit in Iñupiat parlance, alternatively "the good Lord," to whom the healers pray. It is not one's own doing, it is one's own allowing. It cannot be forced but is prayed for; "prayer" is of that nature and is rather mysterious. A nonegoistic intention is necessary, but intention is not it. It is the allowing of an opening.

The practical part of Iñupiat healing is to create a conversation between the two bodies by means of the hands' work. The hands say, "Hello, do you hurt?"

The body says, "Yes, feel this"—and the hands do; they feel the misery of the tissues.

The body says, "Ah, thank goodness you're here. Take it"—and over the misery goes, into the hands.

The hands thus intimately work at the pain, repositioning the organs and attracting the pain into the hands, which are "Jesus' hands." The healers sometimes say: "They are God's hands, not mine." The trouble can enter as far as the elbows, where the healer blocks it off. Then she washes out the bad things she has drawn into them.

When Claire talked earlier of knowing (second sight) and healing at a distance, I realized that in healing at a distance there was no bodily touch, but perception might still take place in a bodily way, shown in one case in which Claire, while sitting in her house, felt the same pain in her own body that was afflicting someone outside as he approached the house in search of Claire to heal him. The sense that could receive that kind of message appeared to be on a continuum with the fine bodily sense I have just described. This sense, though, was able to extend itself until it became a visionary seeing from afar, and the seeing of spirit beings. How it did this is hard to say. ∎

7
Winter

Western Celebration Converted

November 26, Thursday, Thanksgiving Day.
A stormy wind blew, driving snow before it. Under
these conditions the snow did not settle, but left the
gravel bare. The people chafed at the delay in the
coming of hard snow: the snowmobiles could not
run on bare gravel. Even so the temperature was
zero. I jogged in my light, windproof nylon jacket
and pants with plenty of warm clothes underneath,
and I felt fine.

Carrie and I cooked pies for the feast of Thanksgiving, which was going to be held in the municipal
hall, usually known as "the city." We
were warned to bring along paper
plates and plastic bags. When we approached the hall, we saw a few Hondas already parked at the entrance. Inside, the elders were ranged around the
walls. I sat down near them. Lena thrust a cup of tea
into my hand because I was an elder.

"Thanks."

I glanced at the stage. Right across the wall at the
back of the stage appeared stacks of crates of soda
pop and ranks of blue pilot cracker boxes to a height
of eight feet, paid for by the city and also from
bingo proceeds. As the place grew more crowded,
the center floor, protected now with flattened cardboard, became piled high with Iñupiat food: the
people brought double haunches of frozen caribou
from the ice cellars, three-foot-long shee fish with
delicious, sweet flesh, huge bowlfuls of black and

white chunky muktuk, and strange all-white muktuk that was taken from the skin of the beluga, the so-called "white whale," fifteen feet long and related to the porpoise. Crates of oranges stood ready for the children.

To begin the event a large group of villagers with hymnbooks stood forward to perform. They sang in parts, Claire singing lustily among the altos, and Annie in the sopranos. Not surprisingly, they had chosen "All things are ready: come to the feast," and also "He is the vine, and we are the branches." I said to myself rebelliously, turning my chin toward the choir as they sang, "*You* guys are the vine. You." Who else? Or better, their Tulungugraq is the—Whale Giver.

The mayor and the preacher gave thanks, and the serving began. I was trying to videotape the occasion and held the lens of the camera up to my eye, watching the Tukumaviks, the Jacksons, the Sivuqs, the Kasugaqs, the Nashaniks, the Lowes, the Kupers, the Pingasuts, and more; many families were manning the walls and overflowing toward the center. Meanwhile, I realized that while I was filming, my own plate was filling up with shee fish and muktuk, and someone was trying to fill my paper cup with beluga soup. By this time I was starving, so I put the camera down and fell to like everybody else, slicing the raw frozen fish and muktuk with my buck knife. Both foods were crisp, juicy, and extremely good: the frozen fish was like eating an apple that was literally meat and drink. Then Eskimo ice cream came around, light and fluffy, made from whipped caribou fat colored pink with berries and enlivened with a touch of seal oil. I ate it on a pilot cracker. It was an hors d'oeuvre, a savory in spite of the dessert name. The servers swooped down upon their guests and rushed the food to them.

These gestures and those in the Whale's Tail feasts were part of the dominant symbol that I found cropping up again and again throughout the culture, the symbol of the random generosity of nature. The most outstanding of these examples was the whale's leap and its spout and, hidden in this one, the spout of orgasm. The people echoed the random generosity of nature in the scattering of feathers in the spinning top divination; by a scattering of candy over the whale boat before the hunt; in the leap of the captain in the festival blanket toss; in the scattering of candy by the captain's wife during her blanket toss leap; in the shooting of an arrow at random into the air at the messenger feast; and nowadays in bingo, which repeats the random generosity of nature. The ordinary act of handing over something—money for a bag of goods at the store, for instance—was here transmuted into a quite different act, a ritual one. This was nonpecuniary, heightened, excited, and rapid. The movements were suffused with emotion. I later saw other elements of this symbol in the extraordinary acts of generosity practiced at the messenger feast; outside Iñupiat culture it is found in the potlatch and further afield.[1] ∎

I looked at my plastic bag. How did it come to be filled like that? And everybody's, too?

"All this," said Clem later, "is actually the Bladder Festival. They used to hang up a whale's bladder long ago." He was referring to a festival in the old qalgi meeting house in which the people hung along the rafters the bladders of the animals they had recently caught, and then they danced in their honor. The spirits of the animals remained alive in those bladders, so at the end of the celebrations the people used to take the bladders down to the shore and restore them to the sea. There they would become refleshed; they would reincarnate.[2]

"You say *this* is the Bladder Festival? I thought it was obsolete."

"See? We don't hang up a bladder now. Just the same we've turned Thanksgiving into the Bladder Festival." ∎

Now in the city hall the drummers came out and sat below the stage, Clem first. "Good," I said to Carrie. "It'll be the Jackson group appearing today, not the Tukumaviks." There had been two competing dance troupes in Ivakuk ever since the main troupe had been forced by the state competition authorities to divide into two groups. But to my surprise old Michael from the other group came forward as well, and Ed Tukumavik, Ed's brother Geordie, Matthew, Netta's cousin Seth Lowe, and the others, irrespective of whether they were from Clem's group or Ed's. So this was a celebration of the whole, overriding the division into two groups. By now the drummers were seated together in one line, their airy disk drums already wafting up and down. Netta, Helen Tukumavik Pingasut, and all the respective female relatives of each drummer sat in a row on the edge of the stage just behind the men. They were there to sing and later to dance. The soft singing began, "Ah—yah—yi-yah—yi-yah—yah— —ah," light and plangent. Then the drummers firmed up, rapped the drum rims smartly, and called out the same syncopated tune with vividness and assurance.

When the next number began, one woman came out from behind, and two youths from in front. A gesture dance began, vaguely, as in a dream. Then the music struck hard, and the men jounced on one foot—stomped with the other—shouldering enormous unseeing looks here and there—always edging near to the state of dissociation. The woman kept her feet steady in one place, bobbing her body up and down to the rhythm of the delicate passes of her hands. Now at the sharp beat she squatted down, and both men bestrode her in turn and passed on. A cheer arose, for the dance echoed polyandry.[3]

Now Clem put his drum down and came forward to dance along with Margie. We saw him make the first shrugging passes, idling with his feet, his flat face composed. The music became abrupt. Suddenly each syncopated clack seemed to drive him wild. Like a fledgling bird he struggled to fly, kept to the earth by one foot. But his body made it. Quite dissociated, his arms in big mittens rose, rose higher, jackknifing now, the eagle spirit with giant wings bouncing off from the earth, then the last stretching upward. The music stopped, and he seemed to go on soaring.

Geordie, of the Tukumaviks, danced then, a conscious clown, poking and twisting, his eyes starting out. The crowd liked Clem and Geordie both. Then the floor was open, and the whole community drifted in to dance, parents, toddlers—and myself on the side trying the "point!-point!-from-side-to-side" effect with my arms, keeping to the rhythm of the drumbeat, sometimes getting it, sometimes not. Margie said to me afterward, "Good. You're really dancing."

"I've got to start somewhere," I said.

The hour was late. The preacher came forward and led everybody in the Lord's Prayer. The feast was over. Factionalism had been put aside. What dominated was what the preacher called "Eskimo spirituality": in his sense, sharing and prayer. But what was happening was that the Christian hymns at the beginning and the prayers served *Iñupiat* values: cosmological cycling and a sense of the spirit. The Iñupiat sharing did not serve Christianity. The people had indeed Eskimoized Thanksgiving.

Very soon the hall was empty, save for pop cans and cups on the floor. "A superb festival," I said to myself. We found our things. Soon I was following Carrie's rapid footsteps between the houses and through the snow. We reached our own house and entered.

"We've been broken into," Carrie exclaimed. The door was standing open. I went on through. The side door to the storeroom had been somehow forced. Every room had been gone over and trashed. Someone had been looking for something small. Even my plastic needle case had been opened and spilled. There had been only twenty dollars in my purse, and that was gone, plus all the credit cards and licenses, also a bunch of letters. Why?

Last of all, we went into the furnace room. We saw what had happened. The intruders had found it easier to enter through the door leading from the unlocked porch to the storeroom because the storeroom also had a door leading into the furnace room and from there to the interior of the house. They had forced the door from the storeroom to the furnace room, and as they opened it, they smashed a number of large glass window panes that had been leaning against the inside of the door. Glass shards and splinters lay everywhere. Standing in the darkness of the furnace room, I had a sense of horror, of helplessness. Worst of all, the front door lock was smashed.

Annie came in from next door and succeeded in shutting the storeroom door among the huge broken panes that were balanced and falling. We piled up the pieces and swept up the splinters, and then Carrie and her boyfriend decided to go out for the night.

"You can't go!" I said, alarmed. "I'll be all by myself—in a house without locks—and after what's happened! . . ." No door would lock now. The boy relented and agreed that they would stay. Seeing my distraught face, he put his arms around me and hugged me.

We resolved to send away for new and tougher locks.

November 29, Sunday. *Winter Upriver.* Silas, a young hunter who was a member of the Assembly of God church, was going upriver to look for caribou, and he agreed to take me with him. I dressed in all my warmest clothes and my Eddie Bauer down parka with its coyote ruff. I put on some down-filled snow pants and a woolen balaclava helmet with the coyote hood drawn over it.

"Alaqpaa!" said Silas as we went outside to his snowmobile. "It's cold." It was about -15°, and a lively breeze was blowing. I climbed into the basket sled behind the snowmobile and pulled the balaclava over my nose. Silas wore a white camouflage parka that was lined with a one-inch-thick Tuscany lambskin pelt. His ruff was wolverine. The engine roared. We left town by the north edge on the lagoon side, passing through a gap in the banked-up snow fence. We descended the lagoon beach fast and then scooted

straight onto the ice of the lagoon. On we sped into the gray world. Keeping the gravel spit to our left, we gradually entered the vicinity of the river that flows out of a gap further along the spit. All was frozen thick. Silas found a series of small lagoons on the right that were familiar to him, across which led a trail that provided smooth riding until it was time to debouch onto the surface of the river itself. Now for a ten-mile winding trip, sometimes on the frozen river and sometimes dodging the curves up on the land. The sun had just appeared and was a ball touching the horizon. This was at 2:50 P.M. Alaska time, which is three hours ahead of natural time in that region. The land was almost flat, a mere snow waste with occasional stands of old grass tufts and knobby circles that were sites of ancient homes. We often made dips onto clear, dark river ice, sliding down the snowdrifts that filled the overhanging banks. These Silas took slanting with his snowmobile—the sled following at an angle, with myself in it clutching the sides. He shot a glance back at me. I waved "Okay."

It was a land of ice with that mature feeling of loneliness that I loved. The river was sunk between its banks a few feet, so that actual bushes of willow and hazel managed to straggle at the edges of the frozen stream, surviving the blast in the shelter of the banks. At one time Silas stopped the snowmobile and climbed the bank with his rifle. Quietly he stood for a minute, examining the ground for tracks. He gazed far around, holding the gun at his shoulder, pointed and at the ready, just in case. There were no caribou. Silas's unconscious perfect hunter's pose made the scene almost ridiculously beautiful.

I went to relieve myself in the bushes, and in order to do so had to take off my gloves, remove my parka, and let down the shoulder straps of my snow pants. Afterward I had to put the parka on again, which I succeeded in doing. But as for zipping up the parka—by this time my fingers were numb, and I could not get a grip on the metal tag. I tried again and again. My fingers began to stick to the tag. I walked over to Silas.

"Please do up this zipper." He took off his gloves and did it at once, smiling. My feet were cold, but that couldn't be helped. Traveling fast creates a wind, and there was already a fair wind chill.

On we went. After some time three huts came into view on the bank. These were fish camps, now deserted. Silas went to the door of the furthest one and led me inside through the double porch. It was Silas's cousin's cabin. We shut both doors, then groped for matches. I had brought a candle end, and Silas had matches, so we had light. I looked around. Low beds covered with caribou skins and sleeping bags lined the walls. A picnic cooler stood by. Shelves held cups and utensils: it was a handy cabin. Silas found a Coleman stove and lit it. Firewood also lay ready. Silas arranged a fire in the wood stove, then poured on plenty of white gas and lit the fire by striking two matches against each other. He also threw in rags soaked in white gas. Clouds of steam arose that soon dissipated, and the fire grew hot. I pulled a large thermos of hot chocolate out of my day pack. We sat on a bench before the fire with our feet up, drinking many cups of chocolate and eating crackers. We chatted. It was very peaceful. I took out my camera and we took snaps of each other. Silas told me how on one occasion he had gone hunting on his Honda ten miles southwest of the southern cape. His engine failed on him and he had to walk back thirty miles. He told me it took him twelve hours. That happened roughly at the same time of the year as this.

I asked him about the Assembly of God. His face warmed. "It's a small membership, but they really help people," he said in his gentle voice. His cheekbones were high; his slit eyes smiled.

It was now about 4:30 P.M. We were thoroughly warm, so we tidied up, put our parkas back on, and left. On the way home I seemed to feel the bumps more and gripped the sides of the sled to resist each impact. I wanted to cover my eyes altogether to keep them warm, but I decided to leave a gap so I could see out at the times Silas looked behind from his seat on the snowmobile, as he often did to see whether I was all right. Each time he did, I was able to give a reassuring wave. Silas's mustache was iced up. The sun had already disappeared into twilight, and I saw that a half moon hung in the sky, white and silent; now the roar of the snowmobile runners over deeper snow echoed as if there were a plane nearby. But there was nothing nearby. Silas sometimes rose to kneel on the saddle in order to look far afield, then sat down again to forge ahead. There was no windshield before his eyes, so his face became a dark angry red from the cold, although his eyes were still mild in their slits.

Silas now had to use his headlights. By the time we entered Ivakuk it was quite dark, and the street lights were blazing. He let me off at my house. I was sorry he had caught no game. [After two more days he went out again, and this time he caught two caribou and brought me a haunch. The meat was delicious.]

November 30, Monday. Morale was both high and low at Ivakuk. [In this account much material is missing that is too sensitive to include. The positive events must be balanced against a series of negative ones, which nevertheless did not break down the unity of the village. In Ivakuk the good and the bad were balanced in much the same fashion as elsewhere in this world. My focus was not on social conflict, but on spirit perception and action.]

To repair our house locks I had ordered new locking door knobs, also an enormous padlock for the door to the outside, plus hasps: total price ninety-four dollars. They now arrived, and we screwed them on.

December 4, Friday. The moon was now nearly full and would not set at all for six weeks.[4] On December 5 the sun was no longer to be seen and would not rise until January 6. Every fine day we could see a sunset glow along the southern horizon at midday, bright enough to turn the sky pale blue, and quite recognizable as daylight. The glow lasted for a couple of hours even as late as December 21, and it was during these "daylight" hours that I kept on with my jogging.

"Keep a good watch out for polar bears," warned Seth at elders' lunch, laughing hugely. At the picture of me fleeing from a polar bear, the company shook with mirth.

"You're right," I retorted. "I want to live to eat polar bears, not be eaten by them." They collapsed again.

Many thousands of polar bears wandered that coast; they were far from becoming extinct. They often came close to the village, sometimes entering it in search of garbage.

December 7, Monday. The trash man came. I showed him the sheets of broken glass in the furnace room. He lifted them carefully and carried them out of the house to the truck. Immediately my waking dream of October 5 came back to me—a distinct picture of a man carrying a whole pile of stuff like window glass. Again I asked myself what was going on with me. And the awful fault, the penalty, the suffering I had dreamed of had come about too, on November 10 at Bristol. Both matters, the curse of the woman at Bristol and the trauma of the break-in and the broken glass, had disturbed me a great deal. But in each case I had felt the disturbance earlier, in the two swift waking dreams on October 5. Okay then, my emotions weren't obeying the laws of time. I wanted to learn more about this.

8
Winter Solstice

December 12, Saturday. Clem was in my living room, winning a game of chess. He broke off to talk about his plans for the revival of the largest of the old Iñupiat festivals, the Messenger Feast. Clem was promoting its revival at the meetings of the IRA in Ivakuk, and now the proposal had been taken up and supported by the Iñupiaq mayor of the borough. This would be the first celebration of the Messenger Feast since its abolition by the missionaries in 1908.

Clem started to describe how the feast first came into being in the ancient days, and I listened eagerly.

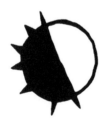

"There was a giant bird out on the Seward peninsula. Those giant birds are the ones you have to shoot with arrows tipped with a special shaman arrowhead. There was once a man who had these arrows, and he shot the bird. He treated it with respect and hung out its skin to dry.

"Then he heard a 'boom-boom, boom-boom' sound far away. He followed the sound. He rode on the bird's back to follow the sound. The bird flew into the mountains, rising higher and higher. At length the man looked down and saw a house below him, with a woman sitting outside it. She was the mother of the giant bird. The beat he was hearing was the woman's heart beating for her dead son.

"They landed. 'I am the mother of the bird who is a man, and he has been killed. How have you been treating his parka?'

"'I hang the wings out every day and bring them in every night.'

"'Good. You are treating me with respect.'

"The man stayed there one year, and the woman taught him many things. At the end of the year she said, 'Now do this: go to the sea, make a drum, and then wait.'

"He went to the shore and tried different kinds of driftwood. When he found wood that made the sound of a heartbeat when he struck it, he used the wood and made it into a drum.

"'Hang up the drum, and beat it,' he was told. He did so. After a time the man heard something coming. He looked but couldn't see anything because there was a mound in front of him. Then up from behind the mound came a tiny dog sled. Its dogs were shrews and the rider was a mouse. Then another sled came up, and another. They all went off for the Messenger Feast, and they took the man with them. When they got near a village, runners dropped off from the sleds and started for the village. This was a race—they raced to the village. The sleds went on and picked up those that had collapsed from the cold. The winner received a lot of food, and everyone ate at the feast. The men brought with them sticks that had tags on them. These were tags of every skin and useful thing they wanted to trade at the festival. They were like what you call an IOU now, a kind of checkbook. Everybody would know by these tags that the men could trade those particular things.

"That's how the Messenger Feast started."

The flight to the mountains on the back of the giant bird, then, was a shaman journey, an account of flight through the air equivalent to the account of the shaman who went under the water to the seals' house. Although the eagle's parka had been shot, its spirit lived because the man had treated the parka with respect. Thus, human beings, by living well with the animals, learned for the first time the prime Iñupiat art of drumming and would be able to beat the mother's heartbeats; they learned dog-sledding, and after that the prime civilizing art of trading. Even the art of writing is implied by the "messenger stick" way of communicating—the Iñupiat "checkbook" as Clem called it. All this came about from the initiative of the bird and his mother, made possible by the courtesy and respect of the man.

This type of spirit cosmology contrasts with that of Christianity, Judaism, and Islam, peoples embedded in hierarchy, for whom God is usually envisaged at the apex of a pyramid like a king;

"man" comes next, and the animals at the bottom.

Clem's account, versions of which are known throughout the Pacific north (messenger sticks were even used in ancient Peru), is part and parcel of the concept of the cosmological cycling of all existing things—that is, the process of being born, dying, reincarnating, and taking on other life forms in a continuous cycle. Here it is often animals such as the eagle who are the masters and teachers, not human beings, who are weaker and need their help. The animal spirits, so the Iñupiat say, *gave* them these arts. There was a relationship of connectedness throughout, enabled by humankind's respect and its perception of the connection; and within such a milieu time folds back, nature is abundant, humanity's continual enlightenment proceeds, and shamanic abilities are available to help humankind through healing, seeing the future, altering the weather, finding what is lost, communicating with the dead, and conferring a sense of unity and joy. ∎

December 15, Tuesday. Dick's adoptive father shot three polar bears. On Monday Jim Agnasagga's wife, Naluq, cooked polar bear with onions, and on Tuesday Annie did the same. I was indeed eating polar bear. Many caribou were being caught. Clem caught seals. Most of the food was shared around the village. Gordon had caught a red fox the week before. Hunters were coming and going all the time, and this was December, midwinter in the Arctic, with no sun. This was truly a subsistence people.

At 10:00 P.M. this night there was a big display of northern lights. Carrie and I went out to watch. It was dark and crisp outside. We looked up and saw the colors hanging way above our heads. They were changing fast, first making a crown of faint ruby red; then we saw them as an arch; then the soft bands of the arch curved to form a heart; then they made a huge corded, twined rope in pink and green with dark intervals that seemed to coil within the coil. Then filaments seemed to fall from the rope and drop upon our heads. The very quietness seemed to deliver a grinding pour of silent power to the earth.

The trail of colored light ran from east to west high up, crowning the village of Ivakuk.

December 24, Thursday. The village was in the midst of preparations for Christmas. I decided to run around to Claire's house with a message and a Christmas present and to do my main running afterward.

Standing panting in her living room, I first told Claire what I had been wanting to tell her for some days: "Sam Kasugaq says you have the Blessing."

"Thank you," she said, moved.

Her husband, Zeke, said, nodding emphatically toward Claire, "We have religion here, religion."

Later, Claire came to my house, and she and Clem talked, sometimes both at the same time. Claire began spinning out odd events and memories, including one about a man who tried to trick her. This man and his wife had been fighting over what the husband called his backache. "But it was just psychological," said Claire.

The man said, "I'll go to Claire." Claire told us he was thinking, "Let's see if Claire will be fooled." The two of them went to Claire, and she felt the man's back. She found nothing wrong with it. But she did find (as she often did) an ancient injury, this one on the shoulder, now healed. Then she *saw* the accident. The man was driving way over by the northern cape on his snowmobile. There were two hidden ditches, or breaks, in front of him. He went fast into them. The second one jarred him off the machine, and his rifle caught him on the shoulder, causing a big bruise. The man drove home and didn't say anything about it to his wife. And the bruise healed.

As Claire was *seeing* this, she related the story to the man and his wife.

"Why didn't you tell me?" demanded the wife crossly.

"I didn't want to. It didn't matter."

Claire told him, "You're perfectly all right. Don't you come here saying it's your back again."

Claire, like a true Iñupiaq, loved relating direct speech. Now she turned to me, still remembering how she *saw*. "You know, it's like— like fantasy," she said. "I wonder if I might write a book. There's a publisher. . . . Would they believe me? That's the trouble."

She described how she broke up gallstones. "My healing depends on faith," she said.

Clem, in the background, said softly, "Faith. We *know* that Iñupiat healing is real, we *know* that our history is real, all of it." He raised his eyebrows, looking around sadly.

December 25, Friday, Christmas Day.   Present giving took place for the whole village in the school gym. The mayor announced the presents from everybody to everybody, and a Santa Claus gave them out to the recipients.

Wandering around to the other side of the gym, I came across old Mina, a woman who was always pathetic, perhaps a little bit odd.

She looked up at me with sad eyes. "My back," she said. "It's backache. Just here," and she directed my hand on the outside of her thick parka to the small of her back. Poor Mina. I could distinctly feel the rigidity of the muscles. Her parka seemed to be thinner than I thought, so I worked on the ache there and then, feeling her body complain to me. It seemed to talk to my fingers as if it was on the telephone. "I'm miserable, help, help." Then I felt her body assist me to make the muscles malleable and soft and in right relation.

"That's better," she said after a moment.

This was a collective event, done through the thickness of a parka. And it made my own back feel better. Why?

December 26, Saturday.   Ivakuk Village did not sit about at the winter solstice suffering from depression or run raging with arctic hysteria.[1] A large part of the time of darkness was taken up with festivities, including eight days of traditional celebration, especially the Iñupiat games, and after that, the Messenger Feast. The continuous celebrations projected the village headlong through the period, as it had done for countless years.

As in the games of the past, the qalgis (literally "meeting house") competed against each other. The qalgis were the two main divisions of the village, membership of which was roughly based on kinship principles, although it included a large element of personal choice. The games went on for four days, interspersed with food exchanges and entertainments.

While I sat in the gym in the crowd, or went forward to compete in the finger-pull (an agonizing test of strength), I saw how each game drove various parts of the body to unbearable strain. The dead-man's carry tested the whole back; the thigh wrestling tested the inner leg muscles; the elbow-and-crouch self-carry (almost impossible) required the upper arms to hook over a horizontal pole and bear the whole body's weight for minutes on end; the famous high kick required one to kick upward against gravity while actually jumping; the neck pull tested the neck against breaking—all homed in on the weak points of the body. Each trial produced a victor who then faced another competitor and was eventually replaced in defeat by yet another victor, thus continuing the game in strings, much in the style of the string genealogies—emphasizing linkage and connectedness, even in the midst of competition.

At this time the village also put on a comic masked dance, which was performed by the local clown, my friend Madeline. The assembled village saw a crazy figure appearing at the corner door of the gym, dressed in a wild skin coat like a man. It entered in rushes, then performed a stomping dance with both feet (quite wrong), at each sally uttering an inchoate yell. The village was convulsed. I wondered, "Weren't some of the ancient masked dances literally funny, especially when the dancers wore the masks with the laughing, twisted mouth—and that's a frequent motif?" I seriously suggest we have been too serious about them.

The Qalgi System. The qalgi system, which came to the fore in the competitions, itself lent a superordinary nonofficial complexity to village life at the games level. The Iñupiat loved complexity—in card games, in their own weird "opposite-whirl" game of yo-yo with two whirlers, in bingo, and in the bilateral vagaries of "family" itself. Back of all these manifestations of complexity stood the qalgi system, shadowy for most of the year but emerging into reality at the solstices. There were two qalgis. In winter occurred the competitive games, pitting one qalgi against another, and a competition of mutual feast-providing, and in midsummer the qalgis held the Whaling Festival, in which each qalgi used a separate festival ground. The organization was not threatening, as was the district borough and the city, both of which were under the state of Alaska; not scary like the Ivakuk Native Corporation, haunted with fears of bankruptcy and the threat of imminent loss of land. These latter bodies loaded the people with modern responsibilities that had to be either uneasily shouldered or partially shrugged off.

The qalgi system, on the other hand, threw the focus right back onto the fun celebrations of bodily games, onto whale hunting and onto the whale spirit that decided which qalgi should catch more whales, thus imposing an enormous obligation on that qalgi to feast the other. Also in the qalgi system arose the interesting uncertainty of one's personal affiliation with a qalgi. Affiliation itself involved a kind of game in the relationship of husbands and wives. A woman might keep the qalgi affiliation of her parents, or alternatively take her husband's. So the question was, How much pull does the husband have, to bring his wife into his qalgi? And for her, Was she going to retain her own qalgi affiliation? There were many anomalies, and almost as many married women chose to keep their parental qalgis as the ones who took their husbands'.

Concerning qalgi matters, the city might only look on and help, not organize. The qalgi system was by nature antistructural; that is, it was laid athwart the present municipal system. It was a shadow or spirit form, a very different thing from the power structure itself, with very different implications at certain levels. Here the competition of mutual feast-providing *was* connectedness itself, was how much food you could *give* the other qalgi. The competition neither derived from a desire for prestige or authority, nor was it directed toward the strengthening of the order of society, but it derived from connectedness itself. These solstice celebrations were not in the process of being forgotten; the Iñupiat were giving firm resistance to the forces of assimilation. ∎

December 31, Thursday.   The solstice celebrations ended with a fearful snowstorm outside and with tribal history told by old Michael inside the gym. Since he spoke in Iñupiat, I asked a neighbor to translate his words. Michael said the events were true.

"There was a man at the old town site standing by his ice cellar. Looking up in the clouds, he saw two men there, and he saw them descend to the ground beside him.

"'Won't you come to our qalgi celebrations?' said the man, but they wouldn't come, and then they disappeared. The people hunted everywhere for the two men and eventually found them hiding under the large stone lid of the ice cellar. The people captured the men and took them to the qalgi house. There the two men sang their own songs, 'Ah, ya-ha. Ya. Ya. Ya-a. Ya.' [Michael sang a complicated song.] People packed the qalgi house to listen. The people even opened the skylight to peer in from above. Finally the two men disappeared up through the skylight and into the clouds again. After that the people caught many animals."

It is significant that the event took place beside an ice cellar. These cellars are impressive places, known to whales. Whales somehow know their condition, whether they are clean or dirty. As for the skylight—this is the unusual path, like a ritual door or limen, the special path of spirits and shamans, the non-normal way to enter or leave a house. As for the songs, they have power to bring the animals. They are sometimes given to the people from some spirit figure. The songs are owned, and the gift of them is probably the most powerful gift known. In Michael's account he makes no value judgments. Only the character of the final event, with its outcome, punches the lesson home—that the man's hospitable invitation to the spirits to join the people's celebrations was ultimately rewarded.

Although these were words from a preacher, they were shamanist, not Christian. Michael in his old age was more a patriot than ever. ∎

It was approaching twelve o'clock. When the hour struck, the large crowd joined hands in a circle in the Scottish manner and sang "Auld Lang Syne." Such was the mixture of cultures. But their kissing was the Iñupiat kissing, rubbing noses from up to down—bound to make one smile. "Happy New Year!" they all said to one another. Then out into the crazy, wild blizzard of night.

Now came a minor change in my household. Carrie and her boyfriend left. After a month I was joined by Marlene, an archeologist. ∎

9
The Messenger Feast

The Work of the Eagle

The New Year

Something like a strong magnet was dragging me into a set of powers or valences that had become obvious to me, yet they were different from usual. For, when I watched carefully in Ivakuk, I seemed to see the rest of the world moving back behind our village. Our world here was obvious to us, and the other world was falling behind. What happened here in Ivakuk was everyday experience to us. Yet it was we who were moving. The whole village seemed to have moved considerably in advance of the world down

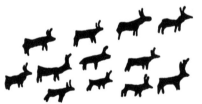

below. Not least among the causes was Claire herself, her knowledge and the cases she described, her showing me how to heal (not that I wanted a career in it, but for me to understand her healing, it was necessary for her to show me), and my feeling Mina's back trouble so clearly through her padded parka; it all followed a distinct and recognizable pattern, but I had not been aware of the pattern before. I was fascinated by being able to sense that definite hysterical "Burr!" that sick flesh in a human body gives out, a signal to other human hands that contact the place and can "hear" the message that those hands must take out the trouble. This healing was immediate, given, and practical; no mental visualization was required because the hands saw.

The next part of my story takes place partly in the context of politics, insofar as the Messenger

Feast revival was centered on the borough, its mayor, and its fi-
nances. Politics were surely wrapped around the issue of the revival
of Iñupiat ritual. From the perspective of the long-term context,
the revival was part of the renewal of the entire Iñupiat culture—a
slow but gradually advancing process.

The Messenger Feast was indeed being organized, and it was
scheduled to take place on Thursday, January 7, under the aegis of
the borough mayor. It must not be forgotten that the mayor was a
State of Alaska authority figure, even though he was an Iñupiaq;
but on the other hand he had a stronger motivation: he was an
Iñupiaq, even though he was a State of Alaska authority figure. The
same ambiguity accompanied many of the life and power relationships up north.

The place of the festival was the elementary school gym at the
borough center. The festival was funded by the borough, ultimately
from oil royalties. The Iñupiat were used to the way traditional and
modern matters failed to fall into neat compartments; these systems
lay athwart of each other, anyway. For instance, in October the
Ivakuk villagers had simply gone ahead and filled the Ivakuk bingo
hall with the smell of aged whale meat, and they similarly occupied
the school gym for their ancient qalgi feast exchanges. *Kivgiq,* the
Messenger Feast, the biggest festival of them all, took place for the
whole tribe of the Iñupiat in a school gym at the borough center.
Clem's enthusiasm ignited the authorities, and the machinery was
put in motion. The Iñupiat were now determined to perform
Kivgiq as it used to be.

The Early Kivgiq. Kivig became a very complex event before its
abolition in 1908. Information is available from the anthropologist,
Spencer, who collected elders' accounts, and from the Iñupiaq
scholar Oquilluk (1981, 149–67), who gave a magnificent description of his old people's narratives, as from the inside. During that
period the function of the messengers on their dogsleds, speeding
from village to village to announce the festival, was paramount; and
their journey was highly ritualized. Early Kivgiqs involved large
numbers of unacquainted Iñupiat. Elders described the ritualized
entry of the arriving messengers into the underground meeting
chambers of stranger villages; the use of tag-bedecked poles, thrust
over doorway curtains to announce the type of gifts to be given or
needed; the appearance of animal dances at these events; the final
approach of the guest parties with their dogsleds to the central host
village, and the race of guests and hosts to the village meeting
house. The elders told of the mock warfare episode that followed,

when arrows were shot harmlessly over the visitors' heads: then the start of the gift exchange, with insultingly small gifts; and the eagle dance in the hall of the eagle, with the box drum hung in the middle and the eagle's skin flung over a rafter. They described the first feasting, the gradual crescendo of giving, and then the avalanche of presents that continued until all the givers' stores were reduced to nothing (Spencer 1959, 210–28; Oquilluk 1981, 149–67).

The ritualized sublimation of conflict made possible the unity of this scattered people, hampered by the worst traveling conditions in the world. In the ritual that took place in the gym, the teaching of the eagle's mother, as in Clem's account, succeeded in transmuting actual competition and conflict into a colorful, generous, and often very funny performance. ∎

January 6, Wednesday. I arrived in a frozen city located even further north than Ivakuk, where there was nothing but a glowering dark twilight in the middle of the day for two hours. The Iñupiat were having themselves a ball, though. In the school gym the bleachers were up, and many ranks of chairs were set out. The places soon filled. Reunions and hugging were going on everywhere. I saw Dora Lowe Nashanik throw herself with delighted screeches into the arms of a long lost Lowe. Helen, Annie, all were there reunited with their expatriate daughters, cousins, and grandchildren.

According to the photocopied program, the Messenger Feast, *Kivgiq* in Iñupiat, was a four-day event. The gym was full. The mayor and the officials of the borough took their places in full force, accompanied by professionals operating TV cameras to make local and state news reports and to obtain an official record of the feast. One borough official kindly supplied me with a translation of the old people's accounts. The speeches of the dignitaries and the elders began. It became evident that nobody was in the least bored, least of all by the elders' careful accounts of their early memories of Kivgiq in the scattered villages of the north. The reports tallied with the general account current in Ivakuk. (They included one account of a man with binocular eyes, who could see approaching dog teams twenty miles off, and this through the opaque wall of his tent. If my fingers could somehow see Mina's back pain through a padded parka, the binocular eyes were understandable.)

The program of Kivgiq unfolded. The seven visiting villages began by performing regular competitive dances, while behind the scenes a great deal of gift exchange went on. Gift exchange itself derived from the first Kivgiq, according to the accounts of Clem and Oquilluk (1981).

I had lunch with Annie and one of her distant affines. This woman had given Annie an entire imported tricolored calf skin for boot and parka trimming, a skin worth two hundred dollars. Annie was going to make this affine some mukluk boots with fancy trimmings, worth more than that.

After lunch Annie and I struggled through the snow back to the competitive dance performances. Netta was there, traversing about on her toddly feet, wearing her most magnificent orange and red Hawaiian-print parka topped with a radiating wolverine black and tawny ruff. Netta was looking after her dance troupe, the Ivakuk Traditional Dancers. All its dancers were in excellent command. I spotted Seth Lowe, old, fat, and bristly, like a Falstaff, with curling-up eyebrows and the crispest, oddest, pokiest style of dancing of all the elders. Joshua also wore his clown-like grin at who-knows-what when his face poked like a bird in the dance. And so did Geordie Tukumavik. I myself began to feel fiercely competitive on behalf of Ivakuk and tried in vain to shake off the feeling. A troupe from Ivakuk must win. The Tukumavik troupe, the New Dancers, was headed by old Michael, the former preacher, who had been busy reviving some long-forgotten dances; this troupe also included the present preacher.

The borough troupe came on first, with the borough worthies sitting in a long row waving their drums in unison and tapping lightly from below. The borough drum skins were made of nylon, not walrus stomach lining. I was shocked. I did not like the gym floor either, it was too highly polished. Shrugging, I went to the front row and found a seat. It suddenly came to me that, of course, this was not primarily a competition for some prize;[1] the villages were there to trade gifts and to perform Kivgiq. Dancing was a statement of the Iñupiat's deep hankering after their culture, re-solved here by a happy indulgence of it.

January 7, Thursday.   I had forgotten I was an elder. There-fore, at lunchtime I was surprised when I was haled out to a huge elders' lunch at the community center, after which there was more dancing. It was the weighty presence of the elders, always remind-ing the tribe of the laws of respect, that helped to steady the throng of a thousand people. I also saw that shamanism was never openly referred to in the new Kivgiq. Yet everybody was there because the shaman power was able to enter through the innocent-seeming arts of dancing, especially in the final box drum dance.

After lunch I wandered outside for a time in the dim light of midday in the town. I saw the huge barrack-like headquarters of the corporation and the more graceful frontage of the borough. I walked by the church and the store and down to the playground, with its ice-sheathed swing sets and monkey bars, and among the huge piles of snow that the bulldozers had pushed out of town, sometimes seeing snowmobiles sizzling around the corner and away. It was not the most attractive town. [The Soviet Yup'ik village of New Chaplino, which I visited in August the same year, was more attractive, though the standard of living was lower.]

At the gym unity was growing back, and as local magazines reported, this event represented a greater unity among the Iñupiat than any that had existed since the abolition of the Kivgiq eighty years earlier. Now I sat and watched the *kalukaq* unfold—the central ritual, the performance of the eagle spirit.

The men brought into the gymnasium a small electric hydraulic lift. One man entered the operator's box and was elevated to the ceiling, where he managed to sling a rope over a roof girder, long enough to reach the floor. I and various fascinated children watched the machinery, but the crowd did not, for such a sight was ordinary enough for the Iñupiat. The drum—it really was in the shape of a tall box—was brought in. The men proceeded to suspend the drum on the hanging rope. It was this kind of drum that the eagle spirit gave to humankind.[2] Around the top of the drum's wooden edges ran wooden zigzags—these were the mountains that one can see inland, the mountains where the eagle's mother had her home and over which the shaman flew on the back of the eagle. In the bottom of the box was a round hole about nine inches across, for resonance. Up along the side of the box ran a sounding rod, extending two feet above the drum. It was fastened at the bottom and center with baleen.[3] The rod bore on its upper tip a snowy owl's feather. The drummer beat this rod with his drumstick, so that the rod in its turn struck along the side of the box drum, making a rapid double sound, very like the double systole and diastole of the human heart beat as the blood moves from ventricle to auricle, organized and timed by the valves: *D'rump!*

As I watched, the installation was finished and the drum swung gently until the dancers were ready. More than a thousand Iñupiat seated on the gym basketball bleachers and chairs were breathlessly waiting. Kalukaq was reappearing after eighty years. TV cameras were set to record. Although the borough mayor and elders did not refer to the spirit of the eagle in their speeches, the dance told its own story.

Clem Jackson warned me to look for the slow drum and the fast drum. And gradually I began to read the dance and understand the importance of the kinetic actions. In a row on the floor a little behind the box drum and on either side of it sat four dancers facing away from us, two on each side—Iñupiat youths wearing orange traditional dance tunics. Their hands were encased in enormous, gaily-trimmed mittens (their wings), and their brows were crowned with headbands set with upright feathers. They wore traditional mukluk boots. These young men sat with their backs to the people, leaning over to the floor. They were "swallows," negative as yet and passive, not there. Behind them again sat a row of regular drummers facing us, and behind them yet again a row of women singers, some of them holding a feathered baton in each hand. In front of the box drum with his back to us, the principal drummer, the eagle, sat on a chair waiting, and another lone figure was seen seated on the floor away at his back, nearer the audience.

The drummer bent forward on his chair, holding his drumstick behind his back. Hanging down the top of his back I saw two wings, loon's wings that were part of the loon headdress he was wearing, and in front of the headdress I made out a loon's beak projecting over the man's brow. A ball was suspended from the beak. [This ball was usually interpreted in iconography as the sun in the beak of Raven the creator, for it was Raven who brought daylight to humankind. Five powerful birds were represented here, the snowy owl, the eagle, the swallow, the loon, and the raven—symbol upon symbol, a surplus of signifiers, to use Barbara Babcock's term (1974). Within the liminal protected time of festivals and carnivals flourish most of the material symbols in a society's repertoire; but, as they burgeon and proliferate, they nourish something beyond enjoyment; as will be shown, they nourish and invite and trigger a special moment.]

Suddenly the central drummer twitched his drumstick, just twitched it: the four "swallows" behind the drum jerked an inch, then stopped. No, it was nothing. The drummer twitched again . . . they jerked, it was nothing. (It was that slow beginning I was warned to catch.) The drummer suddenly swung the drumstick back with great power to make a beat. The swallows rose slightly— and lowered again, for the beat never connected. Their feet twitched. Meanwhile the lone man at the drummer's back came close. The drummer stretched his hand behind and cunningly put a small peg of wood into the lone man's hand. This formerly represented the number of sleds that were expected.

The swallows, although their backs were turned and their heads lowered, had to divine the durmmer's commands. Suddenly singing swelled out and the drummer struck. B-Boom! The swallows rose slowly, turning around to face us as they did so, while the drummer continued on with his beating, executing a mighty swing at every stroke, his hand tight on the handle of the drum, rotating the whole box with ferocious energy. It was the flying. The swallows were on their feet now, leaning over forward and thrusting those immense mittens toward the floor. Had the swallows wakened, had they arrived after their nonpresence for so long? Music poured from the ranks of drummers and from the women behind, all of them led by a woman elder who now could be seen conducting the performance with batons in her hands. The drummer, whom I recognized as Luanne's father, the other grandfather of my neighbor's children, swung and beat and swung and beat, his strong face under the beak full of energy. The swallows kept their left feet firm while stomping with the right, their bodies bent over and arms thrusting down continually. As old Kaglik described it in Ivakuk later, "All the singers and drummers look down, they look down"—and here Kaglik bent low. "They never look up until the curtain goes down." Here in the gym there was no curtain. Kaglik was referring to the curtained door of the sod house, in his youth.

The drummer suddenly wrenched the box violently to the left and beat a compelling drum roll upon it. The swallows all turned to the right, away from him, and fluttered their wings to the right. He wrenched the drum to the right and beat a roll. The swallows bent and fluttered toward the left and stayed there, their hands twitching to the stick's command. The drummer pointed his drumstick right across his body and far down toward the floor to the left. All the swallows bent low at this signal and crossed their wings before them, fluttering. The drummer struck the drum and feinted again to the left. They crossed their wings again and trembled, and did so again whenever he beat the drum and thrust the stick down to the left.

Then suddenly from behind the drummer, from near to the audience, came forward a new figure, waving its arms up and down as it danced forward, across and across. It stayed for a moment violently jackknifing with its arms right behind the old man. The crowd roared because they knew the meaning of what was going to happen [this I did not realize until years afterward]. The new figure took the loon cap from the drummer. The old man immediately helped the figure put it on. The figure took the drumstick and replaced him as the drummer of the box. The new figure was the re-fleshed eagle in its feathered cap—that is, its reincarnation, "its new parka," as Clem put it. The old man left the scene, flying with jack-knifing arms. He was now the spirit eagle. The dance continued in its frenzy with the new drummer swinging and beating as hard as he could. Meanwhile, our minds followed the spirit eagle, that old grandfather, flying to the mountains.

The swallows and eagle faded away behind the scenes. The row of drummers began a quiet theme. They were preparing for the "awakening," the "going out," the "pulling," even "being born" *(aniuraaq)* stage of Kivgiq. The singing began, a jaunty tune with a distinctive melody. A dancer wearing a loon beak and wings stood behind the singers, way at the back. Then he was found emerging, and he was followed by a line of men and women dancers edging out little by little from behind. They made their way forward in a wide semicircle and then around toward the left. Somehow they all seemed attached together; this is because all down the line the dancers stretched out their right arms behind them across the chest of the dancer behind. In that fist they held an upright baton tipped with a snowy owl's feather. Their arms thus seemed to be beckoning and pulling the person behind. In the direction they were going they kept their left elbows bent sideways, moving ever sideways, pushing as it were the dancer in front who was also moving sideways, whose own feather-tipped baton was reaching back almost to touch the one behind, "pulling" her along. So they all progressed, men and women alternately, in a slowly dancing chain, rhythmically linked by elbow and feather, stopping at intervals and starting again with synchronized bending steps. The sound *kii* arose, "Let's *go*," in a low unison roar as they urged still further forward, until all had emerged, slowly, often pausing, then proceeding until they had completed a wide half circle around the drums and filtered away offstage.

Tradition has a secret. It says that just as the last dancer left the dance house, which in the old days was adorned with the feathered skin of the eagle hanging over a rafter, the people heard the eagle's spirit in the skin calling out four times, then again, fainter, then fading into the distance as the eagle's spirit flew far over the mountains back to its mother (Oquilluk 1981, 165).

We were in the realm of the true-experience-cum-artifice of shamanism. But none of these spirit matters were mentioned in the Iñupiat magazines and press. Only Clem, whose great-great-grandfather had been gifted with shamanism and had given his village personal "power songs," as he called them, would talk about them, and then tentatively, fearing reprisals. Nonetheless, we can see depicted in the dance that great urge by the eagle to do the work of spiritualizing, to die and become in that odd way two, the reincarnated being and the educating spirit being. We are here at the very heart of Iñupiat ideas of spirit power, that is, multiple connectedness in the form of a multidestined spirit. ∎

The final dance before we all dispersed drew in practically everybody. I spotted Ezra Lowe, Seth's brother, puckish and happy. I had been told something disturbing about Ezra. He seemed to have something wrong with his leg in a spot where it had been formerly broken and not reset properly. The doctors were testing a biopsy from it. They thought it was cancer. The feeling in Ivakuk Village had become serious about Ezra, for the people looked upon him as a great whaling captain and a respected charismatic personality. I saw him stand up with everybody else to join the final dance. Would he be able to do it? I quivered inside. He walked easily to the center and danced with the rest of them. I rose and walked among them myself, beginning to lift my arms and bend my knees in an attempt at the dance. The event was quickly over. All lined up and sang the fundamentalist "Thank you, God" hymn, first in English and then in Iñupiat, in a roar of feeling. Okay, we were at one.

Six years later, in January of 1994, I went again to the Kivgiq at the borough and found that many more of the ancient episodes had been introduced. This gathering was massive, and included parties of Russian and Canadian Inuit, the former well versed in the ritual and the latter relearning it from the Alaskans. As before, the idea that the eagle dance was in itself a spirit event was officially played down by the borough, though the ancient account was given as "myth" in the borough handout. This time I could piece together the missing elements and participate enough to put them into an ongoing narrative. For me the walls of the gym seemed to open up, and the centuries also, to revivify the experience, which was what was happening to the elders.

Here I give the combined account in a running form, including in the tale the modern scene superimposed upon the old, just as the modern Kivgiq was superimposed upon the old at the revivals from 1988 onward.

Kivgiq, the Old and Contemporary Combined. The feast was always held early in the new year. Messengers went out from the host
village to the other villages, formerly two by two on dogsleds, now
communicating by phone and plane. They entered the village
meeting house, where at first they were greeted with caution and
with much protocol. They took with them messenger sticks, bear-
ing their lists of trading possibilities. Women and men took note
and started preparing fur socks, intricately devised wolf-head mittens, skin parkas, trimmed boots, and many other items, and ordering presents of stereos and harpoon bomb equipment, even if it
broke them financially. When they were ready, the journey to the
host village began.

At the host village airport, the hosts met the newcomers. The
young men of both the guest and the host villages stripped down
to their singlets and running shorts. It was two miles to the school
gym; this last stage must be done extremely fast, in a foot race.
Running betokens a spirit event because these events come upon
one suddenly, not in an ordinary fashion. The young men were
lined up, and at the word of an elder they sprinted down the slippery bus route, through the streets, and to the gym.

The people assembled there set up a roar when the front runner
entered. It was Gabe's son, from Ivakuk, red all over his body from
the cold, seen afterwards mopping his brow from the heat of the gym.

The two parties lined up, the hosts and the guests. Suspicion of
strangers was still in the air, and the hosts took bows and arrows in
their hands. What would happen? The guests disguised their faces
with chalk, so it could not be certain whether they were strangers
or friends. The hosts bent their bows and shot. But the spirit sent
the arrows way over everyone's head. The hostility was deflected,
and laughter broke out through the crowd.

Now the hosts gave out tiny presents, positively insulting presents, saying, "This is all you'll get." But the guest messengers went
forward with their messenger sticks, with friendly letters and trading
tags hanging from them. Inside the meeting house there formerly
hung a curtain, so the messengers would raise their sticks to make
them protrude over the curtain. This precaution was in case of hostility—the giving of a message rather than appearing in person. But
the message promises were so encouraging that the guests were at
last invited in, and the seal lamp was lit—in the modern case in the
gym at the podium, by the wife of Kaglik from Ivakuk.

The exchanges began. Vast piles of goods were on display as at a
potlatch, and many valued objects were exchanged privately. Now

the guests hosted the assembly to a huge meal of muktuk, frozen fish, polar bear soup with rice, caribou stew, and braised seal, topped off with Jell-o and frosted cake. Afterward, the villagers went forward and performed many animal dances. Formerly, strange apparitions leapt forth from holes under the sod house sleeping platform, spirit animals—things of artifice and spirit reality at the same time.[4]

Now, Clem stood forth and danced the walrus as it scraped along the sea bottom for clams, then he rose with his fingers crossed before his face, then with a sudden gesture exposed his face—he was out of the water, breathing! "Ui-ui-ui-ui." He *was* the walrus. The crowd roared in recognition. The crowd watched every minute detail; when I walked in front of them back to my seat I could see all their eyes in a single focus upon the dancer—on the animal.

Frequently two dancers were seen facing each other, their arms in rhythmic gestures of partnership. In front of me, one trading partner had just made a presentation hidden in a plastic bag lying on the floor between her and her partner, and the two were dancing their alliance.

Now the deflected-love dance appeared, done between a person and his or her umma, the sweetheart of one's namesake. The namesake was in a sense the present—not posthumous—reincarnation of the first-named—they shared a soul. So the sweetheart of one's own soul was very precious—but it was also an odd, comical relationship. At the Kivgiq, the person concerned entered the center in disguise—an unknown figure, wearing a hood right down over its nose, practically blinded. The drums started up a curious, catchy rhythm, extra syncopated, while the figure danced oddly, in leaps from side to side, making a crabwise approach toward a particular spot in the crowd, pushing its way past people. The singing rose and quickened, while the figure halted exasperatingly, jigging a little among the people. Suddenly it leaned forward, and planted a kiss on one particular person, the umma herself. The crowd roared with laughter. Others came up to do the same thing, to the same catchy tune—and still others.

Now for the Kalukaq box drum dance. The box hung from the rafters. On its side was painted the eagle, and on its crown were the mountains, linking the borough shore to the origin of the heartbeats in the mountains. There was darkness. The eagle drummer wakened the swallows, guiding them to synchrony of voice and action. This way! That way! At the height of the emergence of the swallows, the curious exchange occurred. The eagle needed to be released from its skin, to be "out of its body." A new winged being appeared by means of the exchange of feather headdress and baton with this figure, and the release was effected. Thus, simultaneously the new eagle body was able to grow—a refleshed, reincarnated one—and take over from the slain one, whose spirit was now free to continue the work of educating humankind in spirit skill. The spirit eagle departed for the mountains, dancing on wide wings, its heart beating loudly, D'rump! Meanwhile the reincarnated eagle in its new feather cap took over its work for the human world.

A comic interlude intervened, with much butt-barging and pantomiming between men and women.[5] It prepared the assembled people for the curious "going out" parade, in which all the guests were now linked together as they left the dance hall to send the eagle safely on his way to his mother. They were led by the prime dancer in his loon cap and raven's ball, elbowing and crouching with the gestures of an archer. At the final assembling of all the village dancers, this figure circled the whole dancing mass of people in an counterclockwise direction, keeping his elbow crooked in the archer's pose. Deflected hostility and the eagle spirit's will thus unified the entire region. ∎

January 11, Monday. We were on our way back to Ivakuk. Ezra, with his bad leg, was in the small plane with his wife, and we had Marvin as pilot, who once told me he was bored with his job. We rose and then flew close to the ice all the way along the coast. Now I could see the sun on the horizon, dead south. The sun! A welcome sight. I reminded myself not to look at it for too long after six weeks of dim light. The plane sank toward the dimming land, approaching Ivakuk. Too bad, there was low cloud cover. The plane flew around over blank cloud to where the beach ought to be, then around again, and at last we located the lagoon and an unexpected view of the newest houses of the village set in two accurate rows to the right, every house banked with snow. Then the houses were gone. We swung away and rose, the tantalizing vision wiped away. We went out to sea, swept in again, and now saw the terminal building low amid the cloud, a ragged, unsteady vision all awry. We rose yet again. Marvin was trying to line up the runway in the fog. We could see none of the runway lights, but only this fog sitting like a neat rug over the runway. Marvin turned upward and went out to sea. This time he gentled in, low, watching carefully, and at the last minute we saw the runway pass below again at an angle to our flight—it was frustrating. We rose up high into the sunlight and turned toward Bristol, where we could at least make a safe landing.

"We should have come down in parachutes," yelled Ezra behind me; he collapsed in mirth. I didn't think there was much wrong with the spirit of this Lowe, whatever his body was doing to him. Arriving at Bristol, Ezra limped to the rest room, which he found to be out of order. We left that terminal and floundered on through the snow past snaking hoses, dodging under plane wings, until we reached another terminal. At last we were all fixed up with toilets, coffee, and a plane trip back to Ivakuk, eventually finding ourselves seated in the plane and snug in our caribou gauntlets and warm underwear. When we finally arrived, Annie's daughter gave me a snowmobile ride from the Ivakuk terminal, which now looked as clear as daylight. There was a pile of mail in the house, and I put on stew for supper.

January 14, Thursday.   I went to see Claire and found her lying on her couch all alone with the shades drawn. She was dull-faced, smoking a cigarette, and quite wordless. I was disturbed. Was she angry with me? Did she dislike my studying her work? Was it something I said?

After a minute she muttered in a monotone, "Zeke's gone north, he's been drinking, and he hasn't come back. He's left me with the kids and bills and everything"—and would say no more.

I sat there crying in that dim place, feeling furious with Zeke, with men generally. Claire finished her cigarette and turned away with her eyes closed. I went over to kiss her inert form, then left. I loved her, and I felt hurt too.

Later Annie came to my house for supper, and we ate a roast joint together. Afterward, when we were talking, she told me about a near-death experience of hers, after her twins had been born. One of the twins died, and Annie was given a hysterectomy in the hospital. She suffered much pain.

"I was in the hospital, and I had a dream. I saw—I saw it quite clear—a house, beyond the other houses, up there east somewhere toward the mountains. A house. I went to it"—she moved her hand as if gliding—"It had two, no, three steps up to the door." Annie's eyes squeezed at the memory. "Then in the door there was Jesus standing! Jesus in his white robe. I go to him. No, I can't go to him. Can I? No. I just touched his clothes"— she picked up the hem of her own parka—"and kissed them, like when he was the healer. And I could talk some other language. Jesus talked in another language, and I could talk it. I talked it. It all came out of my mouth." She bent forward with her eyes forward and mouth uttering. "I understood it all right."

"Marvelous," I said.

"Then I didn't hurt any more."

[This matter of the language was more particular, more explicit, than speaking with tongues. It was more like Pentecost itself. Also there were similarities to a description that Netta once gave me, of her near-death experience, in which she too glided to the eastern mountains and could not go on into "heaven" but had to return. But this experience of Annie's included a healing.[6]]

Annie went on: "Another time I was visiting my son Abel at a distant village. Sam's sister Joanna Sivuq was there, and my friend Jeanne from Ivakuk. It was church time and the church was full of people. I went in with Jeanne. I didn't see anyone inside—there was no one there! 'Where's Joanna Sivuq?' I looked around for her; she wasn't there. I was all alone. Then . . ." Annie nodded upward to the Lord above, "*He* came. Then . . ."

Annie made a gesture right down in front of her. "Living water came down"—she made a gesture of water flowing down and into her mouth. "Living water. In. In." She laughed at the memory of it.

"That night, Jeanne and I slept in my son Abel's bed. We lay awake talking, and I told Jeanne what had happened in the church.

"'It happened to me too,' Jeanne said. 'Just the same; it was living water.'"

Now Annie turned to me, her eyes quiet and warm. "You ask Jeanne," she said. "She'll tell you."

I too was warmed by this narrative imparted by an experiencer, a visionary. It was an example of one major type of Iñupiat spirituality: that is, it was Christian, concerned with the visitation of a spirit, with a dramatic transformation as part of the scene, in this case from a full to an empty church. And it included a gift from the spirit, the gift of a spirit fluid. I could comment that good Iñupiat put fresh water into the mouths of seals when they bring them into their houses. God seems to have done this pious Iñupiat act for Annie when she entered his house. (It should be noted that this last was my own interpretation.) Furthermore, in the old town site lies a pool of ritual water used when praying for whales, so that "living water" has many resonances.

Nevertheless Annie's actual experience was an important experience in its own right, more telling, I argue, than its associated symbolism. That is, the existential fact of her having drunk living water was the central matter of the event. She was sacralized. The symbols fed into that. It was not that the person's psychology produced the symbols and experience. The transformation was primary and originated from "out there."[7] ∎

January 16, Saturday.   Those nights when it was windy I could hear a grinding sound down in the direction of the ocean. In daylight I could see pressure ridges all along the sea ice near the horizon. They got there somehow. In these months the nearest I came to walking on that frightening ice was a brief trip with Annie to the shore ice to investigate places where cracks showed up, and at those spots we attempted some ice-hole fishing. But we caught nothing. This was one of the occasions when my feet became really cold.

January 17, Sunday.   I went to see how Claire was, but she was in her bedroom turned away from the world, just as before. Zeke had returned. I sent Claire a present of ripe pears that a friend had mailed me, feeling somehow guilty—had I done something to annoy her?

10

A Man Lost in the Tundra

The Finding

January 18, Monday. Serious news was going around the village. First, there was much activity on the CB radio. "Dora . . . Mum and Dad . . . northern cape. . . ." What was going on? I pricked up my ears. Dora? "Dad" was Robert, Dora's small, quiet husband with the personality that made him look tall.

Annie came around to see me. "It's Dora's son Jimmy," she told me. "He's lost, out on his snowmobile."

"How awful, Annie! Where?"

"Up toward the northern cape; that's what they think." She raised her eyebrows, nonplussed. "There's a lot of people out searching for him. Beebee, Joel, Sid and them—the Lowes and Nashaniks. He's been lost for a whole day." She sighed and sat down in my old armchair. I went to put on the kettle, feeling cold.

Annie was afraid because of the cracks in the mountains, hidden by snow. A snowmobile could fall far down into one of these, and the hunter would be trapped. Jimmy was twenty-three. He had gone out hunting alone on his snowmobile. Annie and I looked at each other. Her round face and black eyes were restless with worry. We drank up our tea and decided to visit Dora.

I was very upset by this. Dora and Robert Nashanik were the epitome of Iñupiathood; I loved them, as everyone did. While Annie and I toiled across the village snow to Dora's house, we were beginning to pray for Jimmy in that coming-and-going frantic-in-parts way you do about someone else's child. When we arrived, Annie pushed into the house. It was crammed. Old Kaglik (Robert's uncle) was there, as well as Vera Agnasagga, Jeanne, Helen, Dora's daughters, Naluq Agnasagga (Jim Agnasagga was related to Dora), and Millie, the girlfriend of the lost man, faint with fear. There were Velma and her small adopted son Tad and many others. Jeanne, Helen, and Velma were related to Millie. Dora stood in the middle of them, hollow-eyed and weeping, then laughing with her old courage. She handed around tea. Annie whispered to me, "She's always generous."

It happened also that Velma's boy Tad had injured a muscle in his arm. Velma told him to go to Robert in the back room, for Robert was a healer. Robert healed the muscle there and then, although he had a big care of his own. Robert returned from the back room, looking collected. Dora and Robert loved each other— I caught their faces signaling to each other in love.

I was murmuring my fears to those standing near me. Beebee and the others were at this moment far out in the growing darkness and extreme cold hunting for—perhaps—the body of Jimmy. The men went up as far as the cliffs of the northern cape forty miles away, men who knew each hill and dip of a tract that was confusing, wild, and uninhabited.

Through Dora's window the whole crowd of us kept watching the village trails outside—maybe this gliding light was Jimmy coming back, maybe that sound of an engine. We saw two snowmobiles arrive. Two older men got off and entered stiffly.

"See anything?"

"Nope. There's no light now, so we're giving up till eight in the morning. They're sending the planes from the borough and Bristol, and they'll send the Search and Rescue chopper too."

"See any tracks?"

"There were some near the northern cape, and some near the upriver camp. But new snow is coming down." It would be obliterating those tracks at this moment.

Three more snowmobiles came in: there was nothing to tell. The tracks had been obliterated. Dora began to weep; then Jimmy's sister Catherine burst into great sobs, and they both wailed, they wailed. It reminded me of Africa—that high, great, and wondrous weeping.

"Lost! Lo-ost!" cried Catherine, fetching tears from us all. One woman, an Episcopalian, said, "Stop it, Catherine, just quit that."

All that evening in Dora's house the TV was on, as it always was.

It was January 18, Martin Luther King Day, the twentieth anniversary of his death. And between the crises in the house we heard those heartfelt speeches come flaming out of the ordinary round-faced black man on the screen. What came through was the giving of honor to the non-Whites; it also sounded like honor to the Iñupiat. As Annie and I were walking home, she suddenly said to me, "I had a dream. I dreamed about that, him."

"Martin Luther King?"

"Him. King. I dreamt we were in the old town site, in our sod house, and his face was in the skylight. I could see it. Saying something . . . something . . . and then his face turned into God's face." Annie's eyes squeezed at the memory, and her voice became soft, low, and gravelly with emotion.

I suddenly remembered what Annie had recently told me about whaling. The whaling captain's wife raises an empty pot to heaven to bring the whale. What comes into it? It is a "ping," a drop from above, a golden "ping." It is the whale saying, "I am coming to you." The prayer of the woman—is that why it came back to me?

That night I thought, "O God, why do I write notes and not cry all the time? *But I do*," And I began to think about what I'd seen. The women in that house: they as a body were the balancing factor, the antinomian counterpart of the searchers out on the tundra. Were they impotent to do anything about the tragedy? Yes and no. In the domain of practicality, yes, they were impotent because they never moved from the house, whereas the searchers' role was all motion, all effort. But at another level, no. We were praying. Jeanne, the seamstress, gave testimony in great faith; she knew God would save Jimmy; old Vera Agnasagga likewise. Annie was beside me. Before she left at midnight, she led prayers and a final grace in which everybody joined. We were a great interlacing body of women, yet not touching: a counterweight system, just as the whaler's wife assists when her husband is out after a whale—she is quiet and slow in the house to quiet and slow down the whale. In the old days many of these women would have been shamans and would be able to quiet and clear the weather also; maybe they could do it still.

January 19, Tuesday. In the late morning I went out into the darkness, and in the distant southeast I saw dawn break, that is I saw a gap low in the sky break open with a faint gray. I looked at it for a full minute. Later on I went to see Madeline, my earlier language teacher, and we talked about Jimmy and the snow.

"My husband was out there once in the snow up the mountains," she said. "He drove down a slope; then he saw a light ahead. Why a light, just there? He stopped, then he found a big hole in front of him. If he hadn't stopped, he'd have fallen into it and been killed. God sent that little light," said Madeline.

I went on afterward to Dora's and found even more people there, including Annie again. The atmosphere—it was hard to describe—it was stunned, glum, but gradually taking on the nature of deep interior seriousness, until I knew we were in the midst of a sacred event. Robert looked taller again, carrying himself with fortitude. "He has *faith*," Annie said to me. Old Mina was there; Jeanne again; Catherine; Millie and her two children; her sister Grace; old Mary; Kaglik, the uncle; Ruth, who was a Lowe; and her husband, Timothy Nashanik, who was Robert's brother, all supporting him as the news—simply because more time had elapsed—grew worse. All, all of us, were thinking of the cold: Velma; Dionne, who had seen the Satan man in October; Jeremy Cash, the solid citizen; Helen and her niece Edwina, cuddling her own niece of two months old, Catherine, weeping loud and weeping loud—which made all of us weep and made Dora weep. The window watching continued—people continually going to the window, nervous and alert.

A young woman from the Search and Rescue headquarters entered the house, smiling with a deliberate smile. She passed through the crowd and went to Dora and Robert.

She told them, "They've found fresh snowmobile tracks, made on Monday, out by Tuviq in the south . . ." and she continued talking beyond my hearing. Everyone began to look more cheerful. Tracks!

Around me I heard, "He was alive on Monday. He's *driving*."

Out of the corner of my eye I noticed that the TV was showing a Disney movie about the survival of two Eskimo children lost and wandering on the tundra. Now the eyes of everyone in the room became riveted on the screen as the story unfolded. The eyes grew tender at the familiar scenes, at the sight of the familiar animals, lemmings, ducks, wolves, caribou, wolverines, polar bears, and then the all-too familiar predicament of the lost children. More and more people shifted to sit on the floor facing the TV. And they saw that the children did survive; they saw how the parents turned up in the nick of time; they saw the rejoicing and special gifts for the children, including an ivory whale charm, regarded with awe by our viewers. I myself was carried away by the enthusiasm, though still dreading that a mere TV program was no indication of Jimmy's safety.

Robert came over to me (he's really slight in build, and yet a whaling captain). He said quietly, "They've seen new tracks and followed them. The helicopter spotted them but lost them again later. The snowmobiles went out and followed the tracks as far as there was enough gas. You know how it is. They have to keep enough to get home. They'll go back there tomorrow and follow them again."

"How much gas did Jimmy have?"

"Seventeen gallons—a lot."

"What's the weather like there?"

"Good. It's not snowing, and there's not much wind." But it became cold overnight, to -22 Fahrenheit.

I smiled at Robert and said, "I'm praying."

He said, "I think I'll go in the helicopter tomorrow."

"Yes," I said with a rush of hope, for Robert had saved people before in a certain odd way of his. "*Do* that! It would be good."

Jimmy had taken with him a cigarette lighter, a thermos, a tarp, and a good fur parka and mittens. But he had been wearing rubber boots with inefficient insulation. Still, he was young and strong. He had gone out after wolverine just to emulate his brother Sid. Wolverine makes a valued ruff.

Now a prayer was said, and we all bowed our heads. Afterward Robert smiled. Dora smiled a little, though she remained grim and patient. We thought of Jimmy's feet. Would he avoid frostbite? I had an awful private thought: would he lose both his legs? No, no. But his hands would be OK. *If* they find him.

Annie said, "He could wrap a caribou skin over his legs. We try to tell the young ones to do that when they go out to hunt. They don't do it. They should let us know where they're going—and they should go out with someone else, two of them together. I tell Luanne, you should make Gordon take food with him, put food up for him to take." Luanne was the girlfriend of Annie's hunter son, Gordon. Annie was evidently thinking, "What if the same thing should happen to my son?" I was thinking, "What if my son Rory were in a car accident?—it could so easily happen."

Annie told me an anecdote about one of the snowmobile trips she and her relatives made to Tuviq, the next village. On the way back there was a twenty-five-mile-per-hour wind and thick snow. They heard the sound of rattling bones. They stopped at this dreadful warning and tried to turn back—but they had to hole up, seeing that the weather had grown too bad for any kind of traveling. They made a deep cave in the snow and covered the top with their sled, and there they stayed. When they were found, they were so starved that they could not eat much at first because their stomachs were so unused to food.

January 20, Wednesday. We went home at about 1:00 A.M. Annie slept with me that night because I was all on my own. In the morning to my dismay the propane for the cooking stove was frozen. I owned some activated hot pads and used them to unfreeze the propane. After much work I gathered up the pads, reactivated them, and took them to the Search and Rescue headquarters at the fire house, along with my big binoculars. It was dark, with a faint, pale line in the southeast. Eight snowmobiles hitched to sleds stood outside the firehouse, and inside I found fifteen men, muffled up and ready to go. I gave Jim Agnasagga the pads and binoculars to distribute, hoping they might help. The men went out into the darkness and lined up beside their snowmobiles. I moved to let them go, but one of them started speaking, I couldn't see who. The heads went down. I stood still with my head down. We prayed, eyeing the sleds that were loaded with survival equipment, well tied down. The long loads—they were "uncoffins." This scene again was sacred, and there was no question about it; it just was.

One by one the men started up and sped off down the wide, dark track toward the mountains. I watched until their lights grew small and finally disappeared. I was going along with them in thought as far as I could.

This was Wednesday. At the post office I spoke with Daniel, the postmaster.

He said, "If they don't find him, they'll go to that place in the summer and find him" ("the bones," he meant). Daniel bent over the window counter. "The trouble is, young people don't bother to go to the elders and ask to be taught. The elders could show 'em all right, they'd teach them how to hunt safely."

That afternoon when I went jogging, I was in a bit of a tough mood. As I ran, I was addressing God severely. "God, it just doesn't do to let Dora and Robert suffer. C'mon, three days! Enough is enough, you've made your point. You didn't even make your own son suffer longer. God, it doesn't *do*."

On the way home as I approached Annie's house, her husband Sam appeared on the outside porch in his singlet (the temperature was -20 Fahrenheit). "Come on in," he hollered.

"What's he want?" I thought.

Once in at the door, it was IT: "He's found."

God, a glorious moment. I rushed at Sam, hugged him, drew

Annie in; we all hugged; we had the kids all smiling upward; I was
sweaty from running, crying and laughing—we all were, Annie raising her eyes in half-comic fashion toward . . . up there (Annie's way
of referring to the one up there I had been telling off fifteen minutes before).

"Job. It was the trial of Job," said Annie. I nodded. I had been
thinking the same myself. We had a lot in common, Annie and I.

Well, he was found. And alive. After a few moments the helicopter was heard arriving. I looked out but couldn't make out
where it was. I went back in, then went home, then heard it
again—it sounded as if it were in the village. Where? East? Echoing
west? By the city hall? (In fact, the pilot was flying low over us as a
signal before he took Jimmy on to the airstrip.) At home I couldn't
stay put, thinking of the helicopter and—the young man. By the
time I had put on my parka and hood the sound had ceased. I went
to Dora's. Outside her house in the snow it was all quiet save for a
parked snowmobile and a boy on toy skis. I knocked—and entered
a room crammed with people, who turned toward me.

"Congratulations, everybody," I exclaimed. "You did it!" They
laughed delightedly.

"And him up there," I nodded upward quickly before I could be
theologically faulted.

There stood Catherine. I hugged her *big*, the huge crying sister.
Then went over as Dora came to me and we had a big hug—we
were so happy; and I stood back in the glorifying crowd, which had
become quite a gospel scene. "Praise *God*," they said, and "*Thank
you, Jesus*." In a moment they burst out singing to the tune of
Amazing Grace, "Praise God—" over and over. Surely the Christian church was alive and well and living in Ivakuk.

I said to Jeanne, "You see, it took the men out there and the
women in here to do it." That reference to the structure of the village—"men," "women"—left her cold, as structuralism always did
in Ivakuk.

Claire came over and hugged me and said she'd been having
some kind of bad time, maybe because her husband was away. She
thanked me for the pears. "I hid them in my room, away from the
kids," she said. She laughed. "I ate them myself, every one, they
were so juicy." So that was all right.

"He's here!" hollered the children who had been watching at
the window. Everyone crowded to look. The pickup from the
airstrip had halted outside and we saw people getting out.

"Where is he, where is he?" the watchers asked. Then laughter.

"He's getting his gear out. He's there." A young man appeared in a white hunting parka carrying his gear, surrounded by a little crowd.

Dora rushed out in her thin emerald blouse. The watchers hushed. The two were hugging, the one in green and the slight form in white. A hug. We all stood and looked toward the door. People came in, and more after them, then Dora charged forward to the kitchen to put on food for him—in her green blouse, her face buoyant and red with tears. The younger brother Sid came in, and Catherine's boyfriend; Millie, the girlfriend; and after them a young figure with long black hair—Jimmy. There was an explosion of joy, a terrific clap, and a cheer.

"He's walking; he's *walking*." That was a surprise. The young man walked limber and cool to the kitchen—for food, obviously.

"Welcome home, Jimmy!"

"He's been walking since Monday."

Robert entered, his eyes lit up in a controlled face. He went to the far end of the room and sat at the table. Suellen, his sister, was at the table too; Dora's sister Ruth entered, and many others. There was an expansion of spirit; this was the resolution of our troubles. God, god, god.

Kaglik asked for silence. He took up the Citizens Band microphone and spoke to the village: "Godiq . . . ," praying in Iñupiat with spontaneous thanks, though emotion created gaps in his old voice. Messages came back on the CB: "Thank you, Jesus." This was Annie's voice. Afterward she asked me, "Did you hear me?"

"Sure thing."

In no minutes Dora grabbed her parka and went out on her three wheeler, shopping for food. It was known that later that evening she and Millie went to bingo and won $200. It so happened that on the way home I encountered Clem's wife, Margie, and we exclaimed together about the bingo win. Marjorie was an avid bingo player.

She said, knowing I would understand, "Dora won because her karma was good." So Margie had a belief in Hindu karma.

Meanwhile, at Robert's house people were leaving. I went up to Robert and said, "Thank God. And you were right to go in the helicopter. That had something to do with it. You the father." He thanked me—why?—and I left.

When I visited Annie next door, Sam told me, "When Jimmy heard the chopper fly over he set fire to his mittens and tarp and made a big smoke"—which saved his life. Jimmy did not look as if he had frostbite. "These boys are tough," said Sam. What had happened was that his snowmobile broke down out in the tundra five-sixths of the way upriver, about a hundred miles from Ivakuk or any other inhabited place.

Sam's son Gordon, who had been out with the rescuers, now returned with frostbite on his cheeks. He had in fact taken meat and sausages with him. I brought out a map, and he pointed out knowledgeably where Jimmy had been. It was a region with nothing in it but rivers and mountains blanketed with snow. A fog was also over the area, so Gordon had used a compass, and his companion had used another.

"Did you follow your own tracks back?"

"No. You have to head toward the beach going back, then follow along the beach home."

This was at 10:00 P.M. Gordon was sitting at the table, hungrily devouring a roast leg of caribou. He and Sam cut pieces from it and dipped them into seal oil. Samuel gave me a piece. That was strong seal oil. Annie gave me trout from Tuviq, which I liked very much, just as it was, frozen. I myself had been over to Claire earlier with a joint of caribou because her daughter said they hadn't any. I had a shee fish from Madeline to eat the next day. Always there was food.

That night the CB radio was full of speeches. I heard the Search and Rescue squad ordering the rescuers home. Robert came on the CB and thanked the squad and the National Guard and all those who prayed. It appeared there had been seventeen snowmobiles out on the search.

By now everyone was acting cheerful and funny and expressive—almost everyone. Later that evening the following was heard on the CB:

Woman's voice: "When's the movie?" (Sylvester Stallone was scheduled in the school gym).

Child's voice: "I think they canceled the movie."

Woman: "How come?"

Silence.

Woman: "How come?"

Silence.

Child: "How should I know?"

Man's voice: "Sure it's an earthquake on. . . ."

At midnight the CB announced: "All the Search and Rescue members made it home."

January 21, Thursday.   What had been Jimmy's own experience out there?

Naluq, whose mother-in-law was a Lowe, told me, "Jimmy's leg was swollen, and his jaw was too. When he went to sleep on the snow he wrapped himself in his tarp, but one arm got wet; he turned over, and the other arm got wet. These boys are tough."

And when Naluq's husband, my friend Jim Agnasagga, came back from the search, he told me, "The first day Jimmy was out the oil seized up, so he tried to walk to the beach; but he got mixed up, see, and walked into the mountains by mistake. The snow was one foot deep up there in the mountains, and Jimmy was very tired from walking through it. Those snowmobile tracks down by Tuviq got covered with snow, and the rescuers had to brush off the snow in order to find which direction he'd been going in. In fact, the fog was so bad that all the rescuers had to use compasses. Jimmy used gas to make a fire of willow twigs; that was for warmth when he rested. He had signal rockets with him, all right. He set one of them off when he heard the plane that first day, and two on the second day. No one saw the rockets go up because of the fog, and then there were none left. He had a blowtorch with him, and that's what he used to set fire to his tarp and mitts when he heard the helicopter go over."

Others told me in soft awed voices of the dread attending their experiences of being lost or of being stranded on an ice floe. All through their isolation these men continually wondered if they were going to make it.

Now on the Thursday the weather was vile. It was -16 degrees Fahrenheit with a wind chill up to -50 degrees Fahrenheit along with blown snow. I did not run that day. During the morning Dora came on the CB with her voice full of tears to say thank you. She was quoting Psalm 130:

> Out of the depths have I cried unto thee, O Lord.
> Lord, hear my voice:
>> let thine ears be attentive to the voice of my
>> supplications.
> If thou, Lord, shouldest mark iniquities,
>> O Lord, who shall stand?
> But there is forgiveness with thee,
>> that thou mayest be feared.
> I wait for the Lord, my soul doth wait,
>> and in his word do I hope.
> My soul waiteth for the Lord
>> more than they that watch for the morning:
>> I say, more than they that watch for the morning.
> Let Israel hope in the Lord:

for with the Lord there is mercy,
and with him is plenteous redemption.
And he shall redeem Israel from all his iniquities.

It can be seen how the Iñupiat were entering under my
skin and how I was partly entering under the skin of various people—Annie and Dora, for instance—but failed to
do so directly in the case of Jimmy himself. At the time I
was trying not to think of Jimmy in the whiteout, horribly aware
how far he was from home, trudging down some deceptive slope
that seemed to lead to the beach but never did, only toward high
slopes further on. Always "Where am I?"—that totally frightened
feeling. And this was going on for days and days. No. One needed
to be among that mass of women to endure the knowledge. What I
had been exploring was where in a familiar social environment
these barriers to shared consciousness exist and by what means they
are dissolved. When the gathering became stunned, glum, and
gradually entered into that sacred place—was it the courts of
death?—the knowledge could now exist at this blind level, where
all of the people were held, as they would say, in God's hand. Annie told me that Robert never lost faith that his boy would be
found. Robert was known for those special Iñupiat gifts that were
his own private affair—powers of finding and saving. Here was a
level of consciousness that few of us others had entered—but the
big drama showed where that level was. My argument is that anthropological writing can well live around these levels of human experience. For after all, nothing human is alien to us, as our motto
says.

My friends and I were playing a counterpoint of viewpoints with
each other: Annie and I, both mothers, both Christian, with our
thoughts of God and Job and our own sons; and Annie and Madeline remembering past miracles—the emphasis being not on their
words as quotations, as text, but on their actual memory, alive with
the miracle itself, alive too in Annie's case with the dream of Martin
Luther King and God. Then Annie and the postmaster: these two
were sore with the young for their failure to attend to the advice of
the elders, both coming out with the complaint, "If only they'd listen, they wouldn't get into such danger."

Then suddenly there came the entry of the practical—the
woman from the firehouse, saying that tracks had been seen, and
Robert's decision to go up in the helicopter. This was the heart of
the matter—a practicality of that sure-handed kind that knows the

future is okay. By contrast, my own reproach to God while jogging was slight—funny at best, showing my peripheral position, yet with a burst of personal feeling. The boy had already been saved, anyway. The practicality of the burning mitten, and the helicopter containing the powerful miracle worker, were the answer to the window-longing, to the "if onlys," to the time in the world of prayer and the remembering of past miracles; it became too the reply to the appearance of the sacred realm, a realm powered by antipower, that curious power-of-the-weak of us women—which, I should warn, is of all power the least easy to measure because where it operates is beyond words. Enough to repeat that that world is seen as solid when you are within it, a view that contrasts with how it looks when you are outside it—showing the palpable existence of different modes of being.

Further signs of the double nature of the events were also seen in the resolution, in the work of the finding, on the one hand, and the announcements and response, on the other, the first practical, and the second open-ended to what the people knew as "the Almighty," exploding outward until the response culminated in Dora's psalm.

As in most Iñupiat events the two levels wove in and out of each other continually, with a fusion of them at the center, at the finding, in the activation of Robert's unspoken powers. ∎

11

The Grandmother Speaks a *Word*

January 21, Thursday, continued. That evening I visited Netta and found her in her private bedroom down the passage. She began to talk in her soft voice, and for once I was able to tape what she said. She was an accomplished oral historian, and she knew I was open to whatever she wanted to say.

"Yes, tell me about your healing."

She faced me as if I were the patient. "I would never say anything," she said. "Just *see* enough before I cure. I say my prayer in my mind: 'I want to use Jesus' hands for healing.' If you trust and believe, it really works." Her hands went down in assurance. "In the old days it was just like that with a shaman. There was no song. They talked to the person that was sick."

I listened carefully. So the healing called "working on the body," with the hands, was also done in the old days by shamans. [The early ethnographers had documented elders' accounts of dramatic shaman journeys, but not hands-on healing. What Netta was describing was the kind I was learning: *seeing* with the hands before curing.]

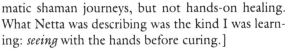

She wanted me to know about other shamanic methods. For instance, the *word*. "If a young boy made fun of you or threw rocks at your house, or broke stuff in the house, my ancestors would say a word only, they would speak that word to the teenage boy.

"I tried it once when Clement was little, that high." She made a gesture. "The *North Star*, the barge, you know, was hauling lots of yearly supplies to the village. Then it was good nice weather, in August. The *North Star* came in and began to haul lots of groceries. All the people worked. I have a book about it, written by my husband and me when they were first raising up the native store.

"Then we were hauling lots of food. Two partners worked together, two women for the hundred-pound sacks of flour. We helped each other; we all hauled them from the boat. And there were little boxes, one at a time. It was in 1940. I should write it down. Every year the National Guard, the army, brought the barge over. There were three National Guards in Ivakuk in 1930. They lived this side of the mission house.

"It was a big barge, almost as big as a building. We were hauling gas drums. There was a *big* airplane calling in, delivering six or four drums at a time to the southern cape. Every time he went up flying again he always bothered us, coming close by us, making a big noise to scare us. There was lots of crying up the hill there. He did it two times, then three times. He came close again; he thought it was a good thing. There were coal sacks piled up out in the open. We were lying on the sand—ah-h-h, there was lots of crying. The plane almost hit people, and they said, 'What's *wrong* with that man?' He almost hit us people. After that I got on top of the sacks.

"I told him, 'YOU SEE IT. YOU WILL SEE IT YOURSELF.' I told him like this. 'How bad I feel. YOU SEE IT. You will be sorry about it; you will find it scary; you will some day receive it too the scary way.' I told him. At first my grandson Clement was crying. I gave him lots of love.

"We brought all the children over to the tent, to the one who cooked for us because we did the hauling. We brought all the kids and waited there. Lines of us were coming in. The airplane was out there, and everybody was watching him. I knew when he was coming in; that thing came in; we saw the plane coming down to the land and then going up again.

"We summed up the stuff and put it in the tent and got ready. We were waiting and hauling. We hauled the sugar and the pilot bread, the flour and rice; we hauled it over on top, and then somebody said, 'I see smoke, black smoke up there at the lagoon.' Everybody said, 'Run,' and all the men ran over to that lagoon. He had landed there; the plane had landed. It was exposed to gas, and the gas burned out everything. The men saved themselves. The pilot was all black. He saved himself by jumping out of his window because everything was loose in the airplane and was burning.

"We hadn't tried to cook yet. Right there they came in. There was no more plane. That plane had dropped down, and everything got burnt. In the water up there [at the lagoon] all the gas had burnt out. The man himself said, 'Bring me home to the store.' He was only wearing a shirt: his jacket had been burnt off.

"I saw him in the store.

"'Are you the pilot of that big plane? You see, you scared us all, our grandchildren, our children, you made them cry lots. *Scaring* them. How come? You don't like the Iñupiat?'

"He started to stammer. *He* was scared, he was getting scared.

"'How come you were scaring us like that? I've punished you, all right. Good Iñupiat don't like to see men like this. You going to do that again?' [Netta's voice was ominous.]

"'No.' [A humble voice.]

"'You hungry?'

"'Yes.'

"'Lots of food in the ice cellars. We've been hauling supplies for all the year round. You scared us. We like to put the food away in the store.'

"'I'm sorry,' he said. 'I'm sorry.'

"'You are not so. I don't trust you yet. How come you might be going to do like that again?'

"Then the coast guard with the *North Star* called the people to go down to the boat. Lots of people talked to the captain down there, too. I never found out his name. I should write down his name.

"That's a hard *word*, eh?" said Netta to me, when she finished speaking.

"Sure is, Netta," I answered. I looked at her with respect.

[Netta told me later that someone else taught her how to use the *word*, but she wouldn't say who. "One *word* only," she said, and assured me, "The pilot wasn't set on fire, not hurt. Parts of the plane are still to be seen out there" (Netta nodded toward the lagoon).]

I wanted to know if this power was mainly used with drumming. "Don't you need to drum to go into trance?" I asked.

"No, not that I've heard of. You sit and sing." She demonstrated by looking afar for a moment. Then she sang quietly and gradually closed her eyes until her head sank down, showing me how it was done.[1]

This woman was not a nice, sweet, amenable person. Her gritty nature sometimes surprised people in the village with its power, and it surprised me too. It seemed to emit direct from the ice culture, like the awful draft that blew up through the sink hole into the warm kitchen. There was no messing with Netta: she was an element, like an artist of the grand old school, temperamental and of the greatest importance. When intending to tell a story, she looked into her hands before speaking; she considered, then let out the story like a pro. No messing, and let critics beware.

And I was to hear her *word* myself. On the subsequent February 11 I heard her use it at close quarters, and I was made sick by it myself, although it was not directed at me. This was distinct from what immediately followed. ■

January 25, Monday.   I contracted the flu that was making the rounds of the village. In the night, because of the fever in my blood and the acetaminophen syrup that I had taken, my brain was swimmy, and I found it crammed with things Iñupiat. I felt I was totally in the element "Ivakuk," as if I were swimming in it, taken over by the Iñupiat.

I lay throughout the day open to a series of numerous visitors. The experience of so many visitors seemed to lie upon my still-in-flexible Western temperament and also work into me. I felt that it was the clash with things Western that gave me the fever, and fevers are rare with me. Now for a time I was more at home at Ivakuk than I had been before. "Being at home" fed the senses I was beginning to develop in order to be in tune with the Iñupiat.

January 30, Saturday.   Tonight I heard the same stormy weather that Vic and I experienced on our wedding night, exactly forty-five years earlier. I remembered the roof ventilator on our humble bed-and-breakfast room that January in 1943, how it revolved incessantly in the wind. On this occasion in 1988 the wind went wildly around the house with a deep whistle, along with a high roar and an occasional weird, thin voice like the sound of a child crying. During the day the whiteout was so bad that it prevented my leaving the house altogether.

Forty-five years before I did not have any tension in my desire to know. I wanted to know, and it was as simple as that. Now I had family cares. Nevertheless, I was here in Ivakuk out of curiosity and in search of the threads of connectedness I was beginning to see. Lying warm under the electric blanket at 1:00 A.M. in this village, safe amid this rich stew of humanity, I did not wish to be anyplace else. The wind was like drum beats, like a footstep in the empty house . . . the furnace switching on. . . .

My knowledge of the language was gradually developing, like a photographic print. I was making sense of it as a result of slogging work. I was keyed to Protestant prayer in the church and shamanic experience where I could find it.

Both were effective and very serious. The people's Protestant prayer merged into vision; Annie's vision at the far-off village church when she experienced the water of life, her mouth hanging open and receiving it, was a picture of concrete reality.

"Annie walks in a concrete-and-mystic world combined in one," I thought. "Like Santa Teresa—or Manyosa, my friend in Zambia. Annie and I walk to the post office; we pray for Jimmy, for our basketball team to win, we wish Claire good luck at bingo. The wind rages; Luanne waxes poetical about her man Gordon out there, way out in the mountains—but he did come back a while ago. These are real scenarios. Will there be money for the birthday of Annie's granddaughter? It's the old thick reality. I seem to hold its wrist and am quite conscious of its pulse. It isn't mine. Annie hugs me, holding *my* body, not hers. She actually comes in here to get the peace that *she* likes. *She* lives and wants. All is coeval with her, and coeval with me; we do live in the same time. I tell her my life, and her influence transmutes my life into something Iñupiat. Then she tells me those great events of hers, and we see how she has wedded Iñupiat religion with Christianity. I have a consciousness of the braiding of reality, which is like the Iñupiat delicacy, the seal gut braiding, a skill that produces a pungent, tasty food that people relish, redolent of seal. Likewise, this weaving of the realities with the social flavor is something to relish. It consists of hard-pressed snow, the store, American foods, skiddoos, big fur ruffs, modest, striding men hunters, elders (those with broad souls) toddling to see their neighbors, the busy young women in jobs, dance enthusiasts bending hand-directed glances in the piquant gesture of the motion dance, while the body is in a steady jig above motionless feet—like resting sex; it includes Robert and Dora and the great Jacksons, all in the matrix of the honored ancestors—the braid woven deep and pungent with flavor. Within the curious seal gut braid they have enclosed the tastiest item of all, a rope of fat, the fat of love." ∎

February 1, Monday.   When I went to see Clem Jackson, the family was sitting down to a supper of polar bear.

"Come and eat," said Clem. It was good hearty meat, like beef, but darker. "Eat the fat, eat the fat. That's what made my daughter Fay so strong." He added, "My son Kehuq's animal helper is a polar bear, a ten-legged polar bear. Polar bear helpers grow to a gigantic size, then develop three more pairs of legs to become the ten-legged polar bears known as *kinig* or *qoqoqiaq*. Kehuq got his qoqoqiaq from his ancestor Kehuq."

"I think my helping spirit is a dog," I ventured.

"A dog!" said Clem, disgusted. "None of us have dog helpers. Fox, wolf, but not *dog*. Does it come to you? Does it touch you? Do you see it like you see this?" He took hold of the salt shaker in front of him.

"No-o. It's more like a dream." He discussed this with Netta in Iñupiat, saying I saw it in my sleep.

"I'm not asleep when I see it. But it's still not like this"—I shook the salt. "But remember this," I said, "I did see an African spirit come out of a sick woman just as I see the salt shaker, with these eyes." Nobody spoke.

I was still curious about the way people *see*. "Is there any difference in the way your great-great-grandfather Kehuq saw the ten-legged polar bear and the ordinary way of seeing?"

"He rode on it," said Clem simply. "Like you ride on a horse. It was real. You call it magic. It's ordinary."

"Suppose—say a White lawyer or construction engineer went down on the ice, could he see and touch a polar bear helper?"

"No."

"What's the difference?"

"The old ones were masters of the ancient science."

Clem was also practical about the repositioning of organs and muscles in tribal healing. "You Whites call it magic," was his constant reproach. He wouldn't call it that. He said the healing was a fact, and the polar bear helper was a fact. Real. A matter of simply riding it. As real as the salt shaker.

He sat quietly, not sweating with excitement, not claiming powers himself. He was following the old religion's observances. This was his own proprietary world, and in his eyes, as he said, there was no reason that it should be any business of the anthropologists, whose theories were irrelevant anyway. He sat sandpapering an ivory ring that showed the whale about to dive, with its muscles humped for the act. It was a masterpiece that I could not afford to buy, but I loved it.

Back that evening at Annie's house, my education continued. Annie gave me a somber account of her son's suicide, caused by alcoholism. "When Sam Junior shot himself, I was sitting here, and Sam Senior was sitting there. Sam Senior will witness to it. I didn't know what had happened at the time. I felt my head pressed down and down. Something or other was very sad, very bad. Then the hymn came to me, 'Just as I am without one plea,' and I sang it. What did it mean?

"The next thing was, they brought me to the clinic—and there it was, it was very sad—Sam Junior was dying. Sam Junior said, 'I love you Mom.' Then he said, 'God forgive my sins.'"

"He went to heaven," I said. I realized later that he was also reborn in one of Annie's grandchildren.

February 5, Friday. I went to Jim Agnasagga's house in the afternoon and ate soup, good caribou ribs, and rice. Jim began to talk. He once told me that when a teacher or a shaman wants you to have a song, you will remember it. When he does not want you to remember it, you will not. This seemed to apply to odd sequences of things that both he and Clem used to tell me. Therefore, I would sometimes have to circumlocute, write around what I remembered; then parts of it would come back, or emerge on another occasion. In the end I could see that the ragged edges of my information did join if I looked at them.

This time Jim said that when a baby died, another newborn baby in the family would be given the same name, and then all would go fine. Jim told me that the baby *was* the dead one reborn. The original namesake could also, in a nonlogical way, be a living person. I once saw Annie point to another of her small grandsons and say he had inherited the soul of his uncle Michael, who lived in the house down the street. In a certain way he was his uncle. Now Jim began to draw a picture of various aspects of Iñupiat life that resonated with this principle—soul aspects that seemed to consist of floating levels knit together by such inner connections. The village could not operate if the namesake system did not exist. I began to see the threads as glowing lines of light by which the village as a family circle was lit. All was enlivened by the paradigm of the *"atiq-*and-*umma"* relationship, umma being the person who was the sweetheart of the atiq—an even more complex relationship than the original namesake one—a type of living-spirit lover. The connections made in both umma and atiq relationships were lighthearted, often of a joking nature, airy and without stress or artifice. The healer-patient link had this same closeness, this intimacy and trust.

Jim said, "About eleven years ago a case came up in the papers about a person who was cured by a tribal doctor. The newspaper's line was that this wasn't so and couldn't be so." Jim was sorrowfully indignant about it. He emphasized, "You've got to tell it how it is, Edie. Tell them about tribal healing."

"Okay."

February 7, Sunday. Annie suggested a walk to the cemetery, so we walked through deep snow to the fence of bones. Annie

wanted to show me who was laid there. Owing to her help I was
able to make notes of the position of some of the graves, most of
which were not marked by gravestones but by wooden crosses
without names. Annie pointed out Sam Kasugaq Junior's cross
nearer the gateway, marking the grave of her son who had died by
his own hand. We stood by the cross in awe.

February 8, Monday. It so happened that Netta had been
to the hospital for a cataract operation and was now back home.
Her right eye was slightly closed, but she could see through it for
the first time for years, and she was pleased. She gave us an account
of a shaman whose eyes were closed. The setting was the old town-
site of Ivakuk when Netta was young. A shaman called Qusaqsuna
was visiting from a village hundreds of miles south along the coast
near the Diomede Islands.

"Qusaqsuna had a secret. We found out he was a shaman, all
right. He was a good dancer. My uncle Runiq and his wife and
Qusaqsuna and I, we told stories to each other.

"Qusaqsuna closed his eyes." Here Netta made as if drumming,
then let her head fall and closed her eyes.

"We never made a noise. He laughed. He laughed for a while.
Laughed.

"My uncle asked him, 'Qusaqsuna! You see your home?'

"He opened his eyes. 'Yes, I see it. They're playing football over
there. Soccer. It's moonlight over there. If you want to see them
play I can let you see.'

"And my uncle said, 'Yeah, we could!'

"'You can see it. I can open. . . .'

"And then that man lifted up the house. 'You can see them.' He
called me, 'Atiqla, you stay by me and you'll see it!'

"I started to cry. I was getting scared. He began to make a
noise, and the house started up, and I was crying.

"He let it down, he let it down, and my uncle said, 'Atiq oquun,
I love you so much; Atiq, it's all right; it's all right; we've closed it.'
He told us, 'It's all right.'

"Then I was almost asleep; I was sleepy. Afterward Qusaqsuna
told us how he saw those two goalposts and two soccer teams.
When you kick the ball inside their goalposts, you win. The losers
might get mad and fight; they might even kill you. They wouldn't
hesitate."

[This experience of Netta's was an aborted part of a full
shamanic journey. Qusaqsuna had been teaching her, and she remembered it vividly. There was always more unspoken in her ac-

counts than she would label frankly. Even I was loath to label my friend with the appellation they were supposed to dread.]

February 11, Thursday. Once a week Netta taught Iñupiat dancing at the high school during the bilingual program hour. Because I regularly attended the bilingual class, I was also there for dancing, among the group of about ten teenagers. Netta, although she was tiny and old, looked magnificent in an orange dancing parka, her withered face open in the same way her grandson Clem's face was open—his younger face. During the classroom session two boys started fooling around. Netta suddenly turned a violent face upon them and cursed them, though the English words came through as a severe scolding. The tone, nevertheless, was sheer daggers. Netta aped the mocking faces of the boys, and they became ashamed.

"The second graders are better than you," she spat. It was the *word.* The weapon struck a glancing blow even at me, and I somehow felt guilty—while the standard of the dancing around me improved greatly.

As I danced, I became aware of a pain in my stomach region that quickly spread all over my abdomen and became a really nasty cramp. I ducked out of the dancing for a moment and munched on five Tums that I found in my purse—to no effect. Almost at once I had to rush for the door to get some fresh air. At least I could go home. I set off, and as soon as I arrived at the house I threw up in the bathroom and felt I would die. I remained crouched over the "honeybucket" commode on all fours until I finally lay down on my stomach in exhaustion and went to sleep.

Luanne, the mother of Annie's grandchildren, came in and found me there. "You ought to go to the clinic," she said. "Hurry. It'll close in a few minutes, and it won't open till Tuesday because of George Washington's Birthday." I thought about this. Then I decided to go because after all going to the clinic was the experience of many Iñupiat. But it was against my will. Luanne called the Senior Van on the CB, and they took me to the clinic at once. I walked in and stood at the service window waiting. In front of me lay the registration book open to the day's patients. I saw that Ezra Lowe, the sick whaling captain, and eight others, including a White school teacher, had already signed in that day. I added my name.

Maggie, the health aide, gave me a regular medical examination with her stethoscope and spotted some gas in my stomach. She went to the CB and called up Claire. I raised my arms to heaven with delight. A treatment! Aha!

I was told to lie on the clinic examining bed. Claire soon turned up, took off her parka, and washed her hands. "What've you been doing with yourself?"

"Here," I said weakly, my hands on my stomach. Claire put her hands on my stomach and immediately felt the gas. I felt everything just as she felt it. It was like turning on a light and reading a map. Claire ignored the lower right pain that Maggie had noted, and she was correct; it didn't give any further trouble. She started from the lower mid-right.

"Your stomach is up," she said—a familiar healer's remark. Position was very important in this type of healing. Her hands were warm. That is to say they seemed big, and the warmth was more than ordinary warmth. Her hands were full of the vitality of that warmth—kind of enlarged with it. She drew my midside toward the front, drawing strongly and gently. She felt around.

"There's a lot of *puvraq* in there," she said. Gas. It did seem as if there were lumps of gas here and there. I felt one lump that was an inch of botheration, and she worked it a little and a little more until it gave to her hands and softened, and became okay. She went back to my right side, doing the big lift action again. I followed what she was doing, feeling the two hands working, letting her do it. Her work of pulling up and forward gradually relieved a lot of the other sore, sick, resistant places full of gas and mucus.

"The middle, up between my ribs, is bad," I said, feeling the place. "Right inside, not on top."

She felt the place. "Have you had an ulcer?"

My mind jumped to the past. "At one time . . . in nineteen eighty . . . four, I had bad stomach acid for three months. They did X-rays and said there were signs of small healed ulcers from some time back."

Claire said, "No fats or oils now. You'll be all right." I was much more comfortable. I rose and put on my things, no longer feeling nauseous. Claire washed her hands thoroughly, as she always did to get rid of the bad things she drew out. Now she had to get back to the teleconference room because her Continuing Education anthropology class was beginning any moment. Claire coveted an A in the class.

"Thanks," I said, and paid her. "See you."

Generally, the hands possessed a practical sense of what the body was feeling inside, as I described before in the case of Claire's back rib. Claire often used to tell what she was finding while she was finding it. In this case she and I followed the progress of the treatment together. It was indeed very practical. Her hands seemed to interact with the body much more immediately, more effectively, and more gently, than pills. They *felt how* the body *felt* pain; they knew it just as one knows one's mother's face or one knows how to talk. It was like seeing. Hands seemed to be like that. One could place one's hands on the plastic table and receive no communication. But put them on a sick part of a body and everything stood out in 3D.

During this February Netta give an account of her *word*—then I myself experienced it. Netta talked about her shamanistic experience, with the house lifting. I had felt—in my flu—the thrumming power that was soaking me into itself, and for which I was thankful. Stories of ancient times, events that today's people were experiencing, and my own experience kept mingling. The slipping from one to another was not too difficult. ∎

February 15, Monday.   I had a new housemate, an archeology student named Marlene. She soon settled amicably into life in Ivakuk.

It was quiet this night. There was no grinding to be heard out beyond the horizon and no blustering of the wind. In the daytime I could make out, way over beyond the horizon, *steam* arising below the sun, vast steam clouds known as water cloud, from an unseen area of open water that was warmer than the ice. It was there that the Ivakuk people were catching seals, like the large natchiq spotted seal I saw in Daniel's house and the one in Annie's shed.

12
The Laughing Mask

March 1, Tuesday. Sam Kasugaq told me that his sister Joanna Sivuq had multiple cancer in the shoulder and neck bones. I wondered why. Joanna was my landlady, a good friend, and I always sat next to her in church. I went around to the clinic and asked if the incidence of cancer in Ivakuk was higher than for the rest of the nation.

"It's always been like this," was the answer.

March 2, Wednesday. The weather was very stormy with much snow and fifty-mile-per-hour winds. No planes came in. I was writing a paper on healing for the Alaska Anthropological Association meetings and showed the result to Claire to obtain her approval. I also left the paper with Clem for his comments and went off to elders' lunch. We sat  down and ate natchiq seal, which was very good. The elders usually ate silently, but all of a sudden they were full of jollity. Little waves of merriment went around the table. Old Seth, with the stand-out eyebrows, looked piercingly for a moment, then addressed his neighbor in Iñupiat. When he came to the end of three carefully chosen long words, he and his listener collapsed in laughter like colliding waves. The snub noses convulsed and the eyes gave up hope in total idiocy, the heads swerving one way and the other, while a cackling chorus went around the entire room. Then silence fell again, relieved only by the gentle clatter of forks on plates.

Raising my eyes from my food for a moment, I looked comfortably at my neighbors, admiring their flat features, high cheek bones, and the strong, old structure in each face. They did not have any stress in them; the people were just enjoying their food.

Next I myself was the butt of their remarks. The portly Seth looked at me and raised his butterfly eyebrows. "If you keep jogging like that you'll never get fat!" And they collapsed again. I grinned guiltily.

Later I returned to the Jacksons. Clem had been reading my description of his grandmother's illness.

"Yes, it's happened before to *Aaka,* Grandma; she's been ill before. Her spirit left her three times. The spirit can be seen coming out of the fontanel like a long line of light. It goes fast. The shaman has to go after it—his spirit has to go real fast to catch up with it and bring it back before it's gone too far. Okay? Once Aaka actually died. She told me that she saw people bending over her body. She was up above, see, looking down." [The near-death experience, I thought, as in Moody's book, *Life after Life* (1976).]

"It happened another time," Clem went on. "Next time she died and went far away, as far as the mountains. And she saw a jade floor spread out, with gold in it, and people walking about on it. They were eating and drinking. She could smell some kind of sweet scent of flowers. She very much wanted to be with the people in that world. But then she remembered her husband, grandfather Kehuq.[1] He would be needing her. So she turned and went back to the world of the living, and came back to life."

I marked these elements: mountains, that is, a beautiful place high up, with people; a place where you would dearly love to be; and the necessity of going back. The Nepalese shamans described the same kind of place, a place of the gods set in a land of flowers, where the shaman climbs a ladder to a shining white house where the supreme diety dwells (Peters 1981, 90–91). Then the return. The story of Jacob's ladder described the same elements. My pastor at Charlottesville had the same experience.[2] Many examples came to mind. ■

March 3, Thursday. At elders' lunch old Kaglik acted naughty when he saw me wearing a pretty new indoor parka. "I'll visit you alone tonight, hey?" The whole room, including his wife, went into uproarious laughter. Kaglik looked at me, his high cheek-bones solemn and deadpan.

March 4, Friday, after a late night. I awoke feeling drowsy and took some notes: "10:00 A.M. I'm half asleep. I've just had a waking dream picture of a room, with some heavy parkas hanging to the left of the door. Then among the parkas I saw a laughing face. It wore a cap and had a scarf wound around it. I liked the face; it was sharp and pleasant. Then I saw it was a carved mask made of whale backbone, quite alive and laughing. I saw its mouth set with many irregular ivory teeth. We were both laughing, I and the mask with all those teeth. I was delighted that it was so much alive, and also because it reminded me of Kaglik on one occasion in the fall when he was roughing out a bone mask for me. This mask here among the parkas seemed to be that very mask. Kaglik had sculpted the original mask face as a laughing face, and what was more, while I was watching Kaglik doing the carving he happened to look up laughing, and I saw that he had been carving his own portrait. There was his face laughing, and there was the mask's face laughing, the two side by side. It had made me happy on that occasion, just like now."

Next: "10:15 A.M. There was a knock on the door. Kaglik entered, bringing twenty dollars that he owed me from bingo. For some reason he started to describe why he put ivory eyes into his masks. He told me how he used to dig for an archeologist in 1939. While doing so he dug up a shaman's skull with ivory eyes set into the eye sockets.

"Kaglik now laughed again. On a shelf nearby stood the mask he had made. He took it up. 'Them's shamans' eyes,' he said, tapping the ivory eyes with his workman's fingers. I saw his face again, with his gleaming slit eyes and high cheekbones, and beside it the mask laughing."

This seemed to be a case of seeing something before it happened: first Kaglik's joking promise to visit me in the night; then the waking dream; then Kaglik's arrival; and the whole doubling of mask and man; and even the mask and myself in laughter. Clearly, Iñupiat found it easy to do these so-called "shaman's tricks," and they were doing them in the modern era. The doubling, such as the spirit presence and the actual presence, and the oddities concerning material objects such as masks, these elements were making play in the episode. Such bits of action are hard to pin down to rules. They live in the particulars, in the details of a real, contexted event. ∎

March 7, Monday. Here intervened a time of fear for the health of Ezra and Joanna. Everyone knew that Ezra, too, was dying of cancer. Both Ezra and Joanna were said to have faith in spite of what was coming. That made me sigh.

Why did I greedily want "experiences?" Because they made me happy. I did in fact experience the snow, walking across the village between the houses, and it made me happy with its curious high-pitched musical crunch under my feet, the squeak of crystals. And the lift and glitter of the air, its electric smell at -25 degrees—it was like crystal music. I saw the weaving motion of people on snowmobiles appearing and disappearing as in a puppet show, gliding on and off. Here was an approaching show, the enormous ruff enclosing—whom? Perhaps Sid, perhaps Zeke. The cortege passed, veered, human and machine gone, seen low-slung in the distance spurning the snow beneath. No, this was Jeanne and that was Luanne, all in the lightsome air, in the strong midday accuracy of light, the great, wide, plentiful light that made me feel I was flying. It made me think of heaven in Dante's *Paradiso*, where light makes the figures invisible, but the rose the adorers make is perfect. No, earth's polar light is better than Dante's. It is all prick-perfect; there is no haze, no confusion or doubt; nothing is difficult to see. All is incontestably there, prick-perfect. Blue, ice-white, the gold of the sun, the scene of houses, they are all what they are, clear. I make a heavy step in the snow in someone else's clean footprint. This mysticism was Iñupiat mysticism, "thing-mysticism," eminently practical and material minded. I remembered when Gordon brought a great spar into his house, which he proceeded to electric-saw and narrow and refine into a huge harpoon, six feet long and three inches thick. The barrel and bomb had been given to him by Ezra Lowe himself in exchange for some fancy mukluk boots Annie had made for Ezra. Annie talked fondly of Ezra. Now Gordon stood like the old Greek Ajax with his weapon. He placed the shaft across two boxes in his house, and he sheared and sheared until it was smooth and how he liked it. The wood was light and very strong. When it came to the whale hunt, he would use two hands to cast it, and when his crew rode the boat up on top of the back of the whale, he would plunge that piece of wood, now worked and complete, and mounted with a bomb casing, a bomb, and a shell, also set with an iron barb—a heavy triple weapon—Gordon's huge arms would plunge it into the tender muktuk skin, the bomb head propelled into the interior of the whale by the sharp charge of the shell, until the fuse of the bomb ignited inside the body and you heard the awesome boom. Then the line running out and running out and at last taking with it the float, large and hampering to the whale's flight, brilliant orange and afloat on the surface—toward which they all steered—now signaling to crews far and near to come and help with more bombs to drag the enormous beast in. All this was implicit in that rough, half-finished spar in the enclosed room under electric light.

After examining the harpoon, I played with Gordon's one-year old daughter, Kara. I took her on my lap and gave her a "snowmobile-and-whale-hunt-ride"; she was frantic with joy and scared too. I wiggled her arms and tickled her, and she was beside herself. ∎

March 11, Friday. It was the day of the spring festival of the Whale's Tail, *Aniiruq,* the festival that would bring the whale in late April. This tail was from Ezra's whale. Inside the city hall the familiar smell was already arising, always reminding me of fish and geraniums: the smell of ripe whale. On a protective flooring stood two massive objects, each about eight feet across, which were last year's whale's tail cut into two pieces, one being the fluke end with its spreading but truncated tail fins (the actual tapering ends having been ritually cut off), the other an enormous cylinder from further up the carcass. You could see the vast cross-section, showing black skin on the outside, then two feet of encircling fat, then the spine in the middle, about ten inches across. Old Seth Lowe was the person to whom all were turning for help—I say "turning for help" because no one "organizes" these events. There are those who know how to proceed, and the workers refer problems to them. Seth, with his fat old energetic body and bristling eyebrows, was in his element. He was here representing his brother Ezra, who was now very sick and unable to attend. The whale was Ezra's fifth of his lifetime and thus appropriate for the feast. There was much emotion. Old man Michael himself, the retired preacher, led prayers for Ezra and for the coming whaling season. At Ezra's name his wife's eyes were wet, and it was the same with many other people.

Dividing this tail was going to bring new whales, that is if the whole of the animal were also given away. All the elders were lined up around the circumference of the hall with bowls and plastic bags to receive the presentations. Seth sat on the edge of the stage, sharpening long-handled knives for the young men. These lads commenced to slice into the flesh, then hack with axes and spade-like knives when they encountered the gristle separating the bones.

Soon the wives, sisters, daughters, and nieces were busy in a work group on the left, using their ulu knives to cut up the large hunks supplied to them by the men. Here in the hall factionalism was absent. Tukumaviks, Lowes, Jacksons, Sivuqs, and many others were hungrily awaiting the feast. The hall now smelled the way a genuine underground meeting house in the old shamanic days must have smelled. It *was* the qalgi for a time.

Kids were yelling and ragging about. I heard Kaglik's daughter shout, "Be quiet for the whale. If you're noisy, it won't like it." There was silence. The whale knows. It can hear. "The" whale is immortal, it is in a way "one" whale; those sentient whales in the sea, waiting to come, are one with this tail in the city hall.

Seth sat on the edge of the stage, eating contentedly. The bowls and bags were filling; this itself was the ritual—the people simply receiving the food and going away with it. I tried to cut off the whitest piece of muktuk I could and managed to eat it somehow.

"Stinky whale, eh?" joked Kaglik. "It'll be weeks before the smell goes away."

"Yecch!" I responded dutifully. We had a kind of understanding.

March 13, Sunday.   While I was working on language with Claire, the CB radio spoke: "Claire. Claire. Come in please. Come over and see little Lee; he's hurt." Lee was three years old. Claire went, seizing her jacket and putting it on as she strode out to her ATV three-wheeler—waited an instant for her seven-year-old daughter, Jeanie, and me to get on behind—and we whirled off. She entered Lee's house, all gentle, already *knowing* the trouble because of her preliminary time of clairvoyance. Inside, the child was screaming. He had taken a jump off the high-up empty stereo shelf and gone crash on both knees. Now he couldn't stand and couldn't walk and was on his mother's lap crying. Claire brought up a chair and sat opposite Lee, with Jeanie kneeling close by to watch. Like me, Jeanie was very interested. Claire took the child's foot gently and turned up the pants leg. Lee's crying grew worse. Claire turned her hand over the throbbing knee almost not touching it.

"I can't hurt you, *I can't hurt you,*" she told him as an obvious truth, in her most musical voice. "See, I'm making it better." She was seeing inside. It was like an X-ray, as she would say; all inside was as clear as daylight. The mother held Lee, and Claire felt both his lower legs. Lee's crying began to give way. She felt down the muscles of each leg, drawing down the legs neatly and together. She worked each ankle, the flat of the foot, the toes, bending them gently until they were flexible, showing Lee how good they were. Her hands went back to the knees. The right one bore a bruise and a big swelling below the kneecap. She placed both kneecaps centrally and pressed them gently into position as if they were jigsaw pieces, completing the action by pressing carefully with her palm. She worked the dimpled areas of the left knee, while swiveling the leg back and forth. Then she returned to the swelling on the right knee. I noted that she left the trickiest bit until last. She pressed the swelling slightly here and there, and I saw it diminish a little. She left that work alone for a time and turned down Lee's pants legs. He slid off his mother's lap and tried a few steps, using his legs like little sticks.

Claire chatted to his mother about this and that. She turned to Lee, "Auntie Claire's going to make some mukluk boots for you. How about it, eh?" Little Lee had been making eyes at Jeanie.

"Come on," Claire told him, "Auntie's going to feel your knee a bit more." She worked on the swelling again, showing me how it was going down.

"See? It's simple." Before my eyes it went away altogether, leaving the normal muscle curves visible around the kneecap. I was attending carefully, having experienced under Claire's tutelage the same sense in my own hands—the sense of a kind of misery and mushiness in the damaged tissues, followed by a similar diminution of swelling. And I had experienced also, when I myself needed healing from others, how the pain seemed to leak away and just not be there any more.

Claire drew down Lee's pants legs and let him go. He walked easily. She went to the sink and washed, getting rid of whatever it was. "The pain goes into my own arm," she would tell me. "My hand gets hot. *Hot!*"

Claire and the mother went on talking. The mother was hard up, awaiting a welfare check. The house was not at all luxurious: it lacked a carpet, some of the vinyl chair seats were torn, and there was only a garish rainbow window shade to cheer the place up. Lee was now jumping from the empty stereo shelf to the sofa.

"That's how he did it in the first place," said Claire. "Jumping and falling on his knees. Stop that." We left before more treatment might become necessary.

Claire had kept saying, "See, it's simple," and it was; it only needed the actual doing. It was healing that was empirical in essence because it was so particularized. The hands knew the details of the inner tissues: they were involved in the tissues, not just laid on the outside. I compare it not so much to Christian laying on of hands, nor to the treatment of the Spiritists of Brazil, who pass their hands around the body a couple of inches away from it, nor to the work of Umbanda healers, with their embrace-like clutches, but to that of Singleton, an African healer in Zambia, with his mongoose skin bag and horn, stroking and feeling and coaxing the damaging ihamba tooth out of the back of the sick person into the cupping horn, and aware of the right place to do it (E. Turner 1992). In both Claire's kind of healing and Singleton's, what was at work was the kind of practical consciousness that Clem meant when he talked about "ordinary" facts. One could term the practitioners themselves, not only certain ethnographers, "radical empiricists" because their experience includes transitive, processual elements in which objects and persons are in deep participation—to paraphrase William James (1976).

It may be that the other types of healers, Spiritists and the like, will be found to operate the same way. ■

13

Preparations for Whaling

March 19, Saturday. *The Weapons Workshop.* The march of the seasons was proceeding. The whale's tail had been treated with respect: it had been distributed and eaten. The whale knew, and it was coming. Now the men gathered in the city hall to prepare their weapons for the whale hunt.

The weapons workshop was an entirely male gathering, held around the conference table that stood on the stage. Men were walking to and fro in the auditorium with a casual gait, scudding their heels as if in great calm, with their legs slightly apart and their heads back. This gait contrasted to the way they walked when shopping, going to church, in the post office, or on their jobs. Seven whaling captains and six harpooners were there, as well as a number of youths and young boys. I was there, hanging back at first because of my sex, race, and age. When the work started, I drew closer.

Ed Tukumavik, the language teacher, opened the proceedings by giving a speech in Iñupiat that none of the younger men understood. But the speech was merely by way of admonition and morale raising. The technical talk was going to be in English.

Ed put on the table a bomb box; Zeke did likewise. Both also brought tall cartons labeled "Smokeless Shotgun Powder," which they quietly placed on the table. They also provided some primer, which was a yellowish-orange waxy substance that had to be sliced carefully, then crumbled and worked into a soft paste. Ed brought a large, heavy clamp, which he screwed to the edge of the table. Other equipment consisted of hammers, wrenches, small measuring cups on handles, wooden tampers, steel rods, caps of soft wood, calipers of a special design, a bowl, paper, and a quantity of finely turned brass shell cases about two inches by one inch. Ed and Zeke opened the bomb boxes and removed some long brass objects. These were about fifteen inches long and an inch in diameter, with pointed tips. They were the eight bore bombs. The men dismantled them one by one, showing the young men what they were doing. The bombs were empty inside. The tip of each bomb was removable, with another removable section below that, an inch long. Inside this section the men would have to thread a five-second length of fuse down through a hole. So first of all, new fuse was run through a tube in a candlestick-like fitting, so that the tip of the fuse protruded up like a candle wick into the top of the bomb. The other end of the fuse, which dangled out of the fitting below, was going to be connected with the main charge in the lower chamber. To make the fuse-igniting mechanism, they inserted explosive primer into the detachable section of the weapon head at the top. As a lid over the primer they set a small metal plate above it. A matchstick stuck through transverse holes in the head of the bomb casing kept the metal plate temporarily at rest until pressure was put on the matchstick by the explosion from the shell below, which shell would be triggered by the vigorous thrust of the harpooner. Then the matchstick above would break, the impact would compress the primer at the tip of the bomb, and the primer would explode and ignite the fuse. The men tested the metal plate to see if it would rattle slightly when in place. Okay. Now that they had that part ready, they broke off the protruding ends of the match so that they were level on the outside surface of the bomb casing. Then the tip, with its inch-long length of bomb section, was firmly screwed back onto the main bomb, using clamps and wrenches. The lower long tube, the main gunpowder chamber, was carefully filled with gunpowder. This was the bomb itself. "Fill it to the rim—with Brim," quipped Zeke, parodying the TV commercial. Everyone laughed, and the tension broke for a moment. The main chamber was then screwed to the upper sections.

The brass shell cases were also carefully filled. They were the size of squat pill boxes. Before they were filled, a previous small plug of primer, sitting in a hole at the top of the shell, was removed, and a new one was inserted, using calipers to insert the plug exactly into its hole. The plug was carefully pressed home so that it was just level, using a rod and something with which to tap lightly. Then they took a measure of gunpowder—about the amount that would fit in a tobacco pipe bowl—and put it in the shell, then pressed it down gently with a tamp. Then a soft wooden lid was fitted on top; then a layer of primer paste was laid on that nearly to the top; then a final soft wooden lid on top of that. The primer paste was sensitive to compression so that it would ignite and set off the shell charge at the triggering action of the strike.

The shells were tested in Gabe's harpoon before the weapon was loaded with the complete bomb. He brought his harpoon forward. The top end of the wooden shaft was extended into a capacious metal barrel about two inches in diameter and fifteen inches long, hollow, and without a bomb inside at this stage. Gabe unscrewed the barrel to insert the shell at its base, then screwed it back on. On the outer surface of the barrel a long metal rod extended up alongside it, reaching some inches above the whole weapon. This was, in effect, the trigger. Below, it led to the lower end of the barrel section. The rod was bent into a hook at the lower end, and the hook led through a projecting channel and into the side of the barrel, then entered the barrel itself and abutted onto a small moveable bar set at an angle in the barrel. Pressure from the top of the rod downward was able to shift the bar inside the barrel and release a spring, which gave a blow to the primer in the shell, setting off the shell charge. Gabe had the live shell readied in his harpoon, and again they carefully checked that the main bomb chamber was empty. The enormous charge was not yet in it. Gabe turned the harpoon point downward and struck the projecting rod against the carpeted floor of the city hall. BANG! Fire shot out from the aperture. We saw then how the projecting rod was the trigger for the shell, and how when the harpoon was fully charged, the shell would propel the bomb sharply out of the barrel into the whale; also, the impact at the top end of the bomb would fire the five-second fuse, and after those seconds the whole bomb would explode.

Gun experts call this kind of harpoon a gun, a "darting gun," that is, a weapon in which a shell causes a bomb to dart into the body of the whale. Ivakuk harpooners did not use this term, but simply referred to it as a harpoon. Harpoon guns that do look like guns are used in some villages. They are called shoulder guns, but they are reckoned to be more dangerous. Even with the darting gun the harpooner has to be careful about kickback. Normally, when he makes his strike, he does it by throwing the whole weapon like a spear at the whale, using both arms, so that he receives no kickback. As described above, the bomb, propelled by the shell, shoots out of the barrel into the whale, and the harpooner can retrieve his harpoon shaft intact with its barrel by means of an extra line and float. This apparatus is reminiscent of the ancient and cunning harpoon toggle head first used in the region in 1500 B.C. (Fitzhugh and Crowell 1988, 123), which similarly detaches itself inside the whale, leaving the shaft of the harpoon safely with the hunter. In the modern weapon, the line to retrieve the harpoon itself is distinct from yet another vital component not yet mentioned, the barb that carries the main whale tether. This is also loosely set beside the barrel, and when the strike is made, it becomes hooked into the hide of the animal. Fastened to it is a thick nylon rope, whose other end is fastened to the main floats that will hamper the whale and mark its position. When the boat is made ready for launching, the thick nylon line is kept meticulously coiled in the bows.

The weapon, when ready, is formidable. It is huge, and the barrel positively bristles with projections. Each of them is complicated, and the proper action of each is vital for a successful strike. The harpooner is conscious that he has those five seconds of the fuse time after the strike for his crew to steer the boat away from the danger of flailing flukes.

This is what happens down on the ice: the men are waiting beside the water, which has opened three or four miles out across the ocean ice. They have chosen a "bay," an inlet where whales especially like to feed. The men make sure that quiet reigns because the whale can hear everything. Their boat is ready, facing the two-foot-thick ice drop-off, a small cliff that they have carved into a gentle ramp toward the water. The boat is propped on a lump of ice so that just a touch will slide it into the water. The equipment in the boat is just so, perfectly organized. The main line is coiled with obsessive care in the bow, the main float near it, and the harpoon itself near to the hand of the harpooner in the bows.

Action is imminent. Perhaps twenty minutes before, they may have seen a whale spout, with its distant roar of steam, seen it rear up and then dive in the direction of their bay. Now it rises nearby. The men in the boat wait until it spouts again before they approach. Just as it starts to spout, they paddle swiftly to its side, the noise of their paddling hidden from the whale by the noise of its own spouting. The paddlers drive the boat up on its very back if they can, out of the whale's sight but in contact with it, to show it that there is some movement, so it will not be too surprised—as they put it—when the harpoon is put in. The harpooner chooses as his target a spot on the shoulder well below the eye, or he aims for the spout itself, avoiding the carbonic acid steam from the spout. He raises the harpoon over his head, using both arms, and flings the whole multiarmed weapon into the whale, hard enough for the barb to penetrate the skin and for the sequence of explosions to take place. The projecting rod trigger, on striking the skin, explodes the primer, which detonates the shell. The shell shoots the bomb casing into the whale, jarring loose the metal plate in the head of the bomb and setting off the primer, which lights the fuse, the fire of which passes through the hole, taking five seconds. Meanwhile, the bomb has reached the vitals of the whale, and the men have gotten away. Then the bomb explodes. ■

Back in the city hall, I looked down the table, seeing bent forms anticipating the process, hands doing the manipulations and carefully following directions. I saw the gentle return of objects to the table—without sudden motion. I saw gunpowder lying on a sheet of paper. I saw bright watchful eyes and heard an occasional sudden crack as another shell was tested. I looked up at one time and noticed through the window the brilliant purple-crimson light of evening outlining the native store and blazing in the sky beyond. Two boys were driving a snowmobile, spinning it around and around in circles on the polished-snow surface of the road, then careening over snow drifts. The boys later entered the center, using the men's casual slouch, along with Dick Kuper, who was exaggerating even that exaggerated gait. As for me, the men hardly noticed me, for they were mindless of everything except their task. This was true education, which connects, the only sort of education that works. The necessity of foreseeing, planning, and careful training was inherent in the very way of life of the Iñupiat.

March 21, Monday. *Skin Sewing.* I heard there was to be a skin sewing party at Helen Pingasut's house. When I entered, I saw eight women over fifty years of age sitting on Helen's living room floor, sewing big *ugruk* sealskins together. Ugruks are large, bearded seals with extremely tough skins. The women were making a new hull to cover the boat of Helen's husband Tom, who was a whaling captain. They had already soaked the skins in seawater for three days, so the skins were now sodden and soft, like wet sponge rubber about a quarter of an inch thick. The proper sewing could be done only when the skins were wet. Without any pattern the women knew which part of a seal's skin they could join to which to form the shape of a boat's hull. This reminded me of the skill of a woman cutting out the skin for a parka—just by thinking, then cutting. They used three skins to go alternately crisscross over the hull, and two larger ones for each end.

The oldest woman in the village was sitting in an armchair looking on. Over on the floor on the right sat Piluq, the second-oldest woman in the village, age eighty-three, with white hair and wearing no glasses, sewing on the floor along with the other women. All of them were in a circle around the outspread skins, Piluq, Ruth, Dora, Vera, Brenda, Agatha, Dionne, and Jeanne. Helen Pingasut herself was busy cooking to keep them fed. They talked and joked as they sewed, occasionally conferring with old Piluq, when they were in doubt as to how to continue. Again there was no leader, merely the use of an elder who was a repository of knowledge.

The seams had to be carefully sewn for the boat to be waterproof. First the outsides of two skins were brought together with their edges lying vertically in front, then the two edges were brought together carefully with a left-over-right overlap of nearly an inch. Now the needle was inserted in the lower surface, pointing the needle down toward oneself for a quarter of an inch, but being careful to go only halfway through the thickness of the skin. It was brought out toward oneself. The next stitch was taken on the corresponding outer surface of the opposite skin to be joined, also halfway through, and the two were pulled firmly together. Then back to the lower skin, and so on, until a seam was made that drew the two pieces firmly together without making any punctures all the way through. When all the outside surfaces of the skins had been sewn, the whole thing was turned inside out, and the second sewing of the double seam was begun. This seam was again done by bringing the needle toward one, also never going right through the skin, but after making the stitch in the lower skin, the upper one was brought up a little, and the stitch was taken halfway through the *inside* of that flap, thus, when done, rendering all the stitches on the inner surface of the boat cover invisible. In the end there were no holes right through the skin anywhere, and yet two rows of stitches bound the skins tightly together. Looking at the finished seam on the inside, all one could see was a shadowy divide and a slight puckering.

The thread was a multiple twine made of caribou sinew that the women continually twisted by rolling it in their palms. They kept the twine waxed by passing it at intervals through a cake of wax. Later, on becoming wet, the twine would swell up and plug the holes made by the needles. The needles were steel, though before contact they were made of walrus ivory.

Only older women were considered skilled enough for this task. Its faultless performance was obviously a matter of life and death because the safety of the men depended on not having a leaky boat. In the room where the women sewed, the TV was on all the time, but nobody watched it. Curiously enough, it showed a surgeon performing microsurgery with needles on the arteries of the heart— also a life-and-death task involving the joining of organic tissue.

The women were not close family members but were self-selected by age and experience from the whole village. The same group would go on request to other captains' households to do their skin sewing. Each woman charged fifty dollars for the task. They talked incessantly while they worked, they shifted, looked for their small ulus to cut thread, held up thread ends to thread their needles, bent to work, and thoroughly enjoyed the gossip, sprawled on the floor with their buddies.

So the whaling season began. Annie and I were already in cahoots, planning purchases of extra thermoses, metal soup bowls, and big food orders from town. It was taken for granted that I would be on Annie's crew as assistant cook. Both of us, being middle-aged women, took a deep pleasure in working on the preparations. Others in our crew did their part, referring to Annie, Sam, and Gordon when they needed information. Sam acted with a touch more authoritarianism than other Iñupiat because of his previous position in the army and because he had been mayor of the city under the state.

The village was becoming polarized to this one great interest, the coming of the whales. The hunt was both extremely practical and spirit oriented.

But the Christian feast of Easter intervened, a visionary occasion in itself.

April 3, Easter Sunday. The church was packed. An old woman carried the cross up to the altar, stepping very slowly— which started the emotion on its way. Ten children were baptized, including three children of Clem Jackson, practitioner of the old religion. Clem was actually present, for once. The first hymn was all about flowers and trees with their leaves, suitable for Easter in Western Christian countries. As for us in Ivakuk, we were a hundred miles north of the tree line. There were no leaves or flowers around us, only snow. But there was light—sunlight blazing through the windows.

I was sitting next to Joanna, as I always did. We went up to take communion, Joanna walking behind me. I turned after receiving and walked back to my pew. After a moment Joanna returned from her communion, tears running down her face. I tenderly touched her good hand to comfort her.

"What is it?"

"I saw Paula, Paula, up there!" she whispered. She pointed up to the sanctuary.

"Oh Joanna!" I said holding my chin in amazement, gazing at empty space. Paula Tukumavik was her sister, dead now for many years. "Why, that's good, Joanna." So Paula was not gone forever.

April 5, Tuesday. (Here I jump back to politics—so the round of life goes.) This afternoon the Ivakuk Native Corporation held its annual business meeting. The shareholders of the corporation, that is, the whole village, gathered in the school gym for the meeting. All sorts of anomalies immediately became apparent. The table for the directors was too far from the members who had to be seated on the bleachers and too far for the tape recorders to pick up what was said by the shareholders. In fact the table seemed to be stationed halfway across the gym. In the other half of the gym kids were yelling and screaming at their games so that most of the older shareholders could not hear a word of the proceedings.

Furthermore, votes for the slated candidates had already been taken. Apparently the papers had been originally circulated by mail. The directors sitting at the table were Norman Agnasagga, the existing president, and Gabe, an elderly Iñupiaq. Also, the White corporation manager, named Angelford, sat at the center of the table with an air of being in control, along with a couple of other senior Iñupiak. Behind them sat a White lawyer and the Iñupiaq corporation secretary.

First on the agenda came the president's report, whereupon my good friend Micky Hoffman, the Iñupiaq radical and self-taught lawyer hitherto employed by the corporation, the man with the small beard and the nervous eyes, asked a sticky question from the floor.

"It's come to my notice that there's a danger of the Iñupiat using their land as collateral for loans. Unwary Natives could lose their land if the loans aren't paid. And the *nuna*, the land, is all they have."

Claire added from the floor, "Yes, we need to protect ourselves from that."

Micky's point was his first move in what turned out to be a skillful chess game against the Whites. Immediately Angelford started berating the Iñupiat for getting into Chapter 11, and he blamed Micky. He warned them that the corporation owed $5 million, which was why the corporation was required by the bankruptcy judge to utilize the services of a White manager.

I became very disturbed. I could hardly listen to Angelford, with his plonking White voice, so different from the habitually modest voices of the Iñupiat. I decided, on behalf of the Iñupiat, to turn to my spirit helper down in the tunnel. I shut my eyes. The tunnel happened. I encountered a strange and loathly object, prickly-shelled, black, and leggy. I let happen what would happen. The dog seemed to have turned up, and he bodily carried me around the object to safety. We went on. I realized that the dog and I had coalesced, thoroughly and completely. Now I was back and watching the meeting. Everything was highly lit, sharp and good to see, of clear significance as if I were wearing extra powerful glasses, although I was not wearing my glasses. The sort of conversation with my dog that I usually had on this kind of trip took place:

He said, "Don't interfere."

"But will it work?"

"Shut up, it's not for you to ask."

I was content to shut up because the coalescence with the dog held. The matter was out of my hands, and I was quite safe.

At this point the meeting temporarily adjourned. When we returned after the break, Agatha, the adoptive mother of Dick, came forward and told the board that they had done very well. Ed Tuku-mavik on the other hand, rose and claimed fraud. The precirculated report, including the slate and the prevoted ballot forms, had totally omitted reference to the land question, which had been brought up in advance by Micky to make sure it would not be missed. The director's explanation was that the first set of reports and ballot papers had been blown away by the wind, so the director issued a second set of papers. The second set happened to lack any reference to the land question.

"Was that a fair election?" asked Ed. "Is the board legally elected?"

The question was passed over, as were other questions about the dropping of two candidates without explanation.

"Your corporation," said Angelford in a headmaster-to-bad-boy scolding tone, "is in Chapter 11. The law requires a proven compe-tent manager to be appointed. You have no choice. In my judg-ment it would be too costly for the corporation to investigate any of these allegations."

Micky rose and made an announcement. "The Bureau of Indian Affairs is going to supply land deeds to the Iñupiat in a few months," he said. "I applied to stand for the corporation board myself, but my application mysteriously got lost. I'm no longer paid for legal services because they say I 'bring in no money.' I ac-tually save the corporation money." [True, the economy of Ivakuk did not bring in any money: its economy was subsistence hunting. There was nothing but wild nature out there.] "Okay," Micky con-tinued, "I'll go on giving my services free." The whole audience thundered applause.

Ed's wife said, "Let's get rid of the White manager and give Micky the job!" Her voice rose and she grew angry. "What does Angelford want, buying cars at the corporation's expense? Let's save the money and pay Micky!" There were wild cheers.

So positive statements were being made. Micky had performed a quietly dramatic self-sacrificial act and received huge spontaneous acclaim. I sat dumbfounded. I had no idea the Tukumaviks would fight for him, that the whole village backed him, that a person do-ing something for free was appreciated. People did know what jus-tice was. Also the meeting was quite savagely pro-Iñupiat, and whatever the outcome, all had experienced the feeling. [The out-come, as I saw in succeeding years, was that the corporation did gradually extricate itself from Chapter 11, owing to the better man-agement of the store.]

April 6, Wednesday.   I was walking by the church when a snowmobile drove up rapidly on my right with a boat gliding be-hind on a sled. The boat was covered with a new white sealskin hull and was escorted by a number of men in their best ruffs and parkas, who turned out to be whaling captains. When they reached the church, they lifted the boat off, turned it on its side, and inched it through the church door, then on through the inner door—as we followed—and up the aisle, and in a trice had it perched on a cou-ple of up-ended sleds in the middle of the sanctuary. They arranged in the boat a large inflated spotted-seal float, the boat paddles, which they set upright, and the big harpoon that Gordon had made, with its barrel pointing forward and to the left.

"Everyone has put in something," said Robert Nashanik at my side. "The boat is the preacher's. He's captaining a crew as well."

Now the captains went to each side and occupied the choir stalls, and the preacher, the small Iñupiaq of deep and solemn sentiment, came forward in his surplice and announced the hymns. The schoolteacher organist was ready at hand. We sang, "Oh God, our help in ages past," "Eternal Father strong to save, Whose arm hath bound the restless wave," "All things are ready, Come to the feast," "Praise God" (to the tune of "Amazing Grace"), and the Creation Psalm, "Ye whales, and all ye that move in the waters, Praise Him and magnify Him for ever." Gabe, Ezra (looking a little pale), Agatha, and Sam read the lessons (one of which was from St. Paul's letters); they read lovingly, in serious, musical voices, saying that all creation and God were one. They sang their favorite psalm in Iñupiat, the preacher blessed the boat, the gun, and the paddles, and that was it. At the back everyone was handshaking and kissing and wishing each other "Peace of God" and "Good hunting." Sam retrieved Gordon's harpoon. They brought the boat out and went off with it on the snowmobile sled.

14

The Bowhead Whale

Balaena Mysticetus

April 10, Sunday. During this month every-one was waiting for the north wind to blow more of the ice away from the south shore into the warm current that was producing open water perhaps ten miles out, too far away for the hunters. When the north wind arrived, the hunters would be able to see water clouds on this side of the horizon, and then they would go down on their snowmobiles and find the water within reasonable distance. Eventually the wind did turn north, and there was water. The next question was, would there be whales?

Whether there would be whales for the Kasugaq family depended on a concern of Annie's. This was her "cold storage." The cold storage was her cave-like ice cellar in the permafrost, located on the northern edge of the 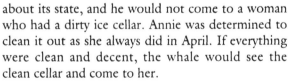 ocean among the old village sod houses at the point. The cave was smelly, fouled with stale meat. The whale would know about its state, and he would not come to a woman who had a dirty ice cellar. Annie was determined to clean it out as she always did in April. If everything were clean and decent, the whale would see the clean cellar and come to her.

I said I would help her clean it. Sam said, "That'll be real stinky. You don't want to go down there."

"I've been in those bathrooms in India. Believe me. . . ."

"Okay, okay, the cold store isn't as bad as that."

So I was given permission to go. I went home and put on old clothes and joined them, riding on the sled behind the snowmobile, in a space beside the tools, kneeling because I couldn't get into any other position.

We reached the north shore about a mile from the end of the beach, in an area where a number of mounds indicated that there were chambers underneath. We stopped at Annie's mound.

"Look at what that stupid Gabe has done!" said Annie. "He's flung all his muck outside the door of my cold store. Acting funny with me! And look, my son Eugene wants to be in his crew, not mine. Too bad. And my nephew too. What's the matter with people?" I felt bad for Annie. However, she could rely on two of her own sons, and she had two other good crewmen in mind, as well as a boy to do chores. Perhaps my friend Louis would join her crew. Obviously Annie was the recruiter. In so many ways she was captain: "The woman catches the whale."

Annie went over to the hatchway on top of her mound and opened it. A smell came out, but it was only the old, familiar smell of aged whale, basically a smell of nourishment. Inside the hatch there was a ladder going down, made of whale scapulas.

"My grandmother used to clean out this cellar," said Annie.

"This very one?"

"Yes." I touched the whale scapula at the entrance with respect.

We climbed down inside. The place reminded me of a sepulchre with rounded and ancient walls. There was a further cave inside, off to the right and further down. There were other echoes of the self-sacrificial whale: we were clearing the way for its coming as if for the Messiah: and also in my mind arose echoes of cleaning away all traces of *chometz* leaven before Passover, a task in which I had also participated in my time.

We worked hard on that cellar. I was sweating and constantly pushed the hair out of my eyes with a greasy hand. Marlene joined us and helped too, taking turns when I was tired. We needed spades to hack beneath the frozen-in slabs of whale, picks to lever them out, and sometimes hammers and chisels to get below them. Annie, though stout, got herself into the narrower side cave and from there quickly tossed up toward us various two-foot blocks of fat. She could work five times harder than I.

We stopped for a break of hot chocolate.

"The whale is different," said Annie. "It knows, it talks to other whales, it knows if you are a good person—it knows if there is no quarreling. Sam blesses the boat when it's loaded up and we're all ready to go down on the ice. Sam leads the prayer, and we pray for a peaceful and safe whale hunt."

She said all this so earnestly that it brought tears to my eyes. The whale chooses its beneficiary. It relates.

At the end of the day the ice cellar was not perfectly clean, but we had done a great deal to prepare for the feast food to come. ["All things are ready: come to the feast. Leave all your cares and woes behind" was the hymn chosen for the blessing of the boat in the church. The words had a quadruple meaning. There was the literal sense of getting things ready for a feast and calling the guests to it. Second, it was a metaphor for Jesus' call to his followers to join him at communion, that tiny feast of the sacrament. Then further, the fact that the hymn was chosen for the whaling season literally indicated the feast to come, the feast of whale meat. But that feast day had not yet arrived, so the song meant Ivakuk whales in potentia, symbolic whales—who had calling power in themselves. It is instructive that those, such as the hymn writers, who create symbolic verses—or the creators of any kind of art—may have their work reinterpreted as literal and thus see it receive a booster charge from some later type of utilization.]

After we finished our work, my clothes stank, and even my hair, now ropy and matted in front. I had enjoyed the day, and I rode back on the sled seated on top of plastic bags of old meat, holding onto ropes for dear life.

When we reached home, I went to the laundromat where the village showers were located, and showered and soaped from top to toe. Back at the Kasugaq house, Luanne had cooked caribou, ground beef, and potatoes in quantity, and the whole crew, eighteen of us, fell to eagerly. Ancient Michael presided and gave the history of old ice cellars in an oratorial voice, gasping and blinking and quite deaf, without much English. Meanwhile, the men prepared their weapons. Everything had to be absolutely clean: the wooden paddles were scraped until they looked white, and the sealskin hull of the boat was soaked until it was white before it was put on. For the whale can smell and see a long way. It knows. It likes to see clean, white things. You feel it is there in the village with you.

April 11, Monday. Nicholas Jones, from the London BBC, turned up in my house accompanied by a load of equipment; he was planning to film the whale hunt. He explained that the local head of the Alaska Eskimo Whaling Commission (this was Zeke, Claire's husband) had said I would put him up. So I had to do it. It so happened that the same evening a large crowd of children came to my house for treats. I was going to turn many of them out, fearing that my landlady might not like so many children running about in her house. But Claire was visiting at the time, and she said, "If you shut a kid out of your house, the whale won't come." The kids grew wilder and wilder and broke something inside Joanna's old armchair rocker. My only resort was to organize them to help make a macaroni salad for the whaling crew.

Meanwhile, Annie was finalizing her crew list, having chosen most of her family, that is, Gordon as harpooner, his two brothers, the sisters to help, family spouses, some cousins and nephews, an older respected man [who later became mayor] and his son Sol, and some almost unrelated people picked from the families who were not running a boat. Annie did ask Louis, and he came. The family ties involved were bilateral as always.

April 12, Tuesday.   That afternoon ten whales went by, causing the town to rise in a ferment of preparation. Marlene and I took the macaroni salad to Annie's and knocked, reporting for duty as cooks in her crew.

"Don't knock," said Sam. "Crew is family."

Soon we were ready, and everyone gathered outside around the boat as it stood on its sled, roped down and loaded with grub box, stove, tent, and equipment. The skin of the boat was bleached to a fine pale yellow. Sam went to the bow of the boat, and we stood all around it with our hands on the gunwale. We lowered our heads. Sam spoke.

"Now we're all going down on the ice, and we'll be making a camp, and this crew will be together for many days; and we'll be good, speak good words to each other, and we'll help. If there's anything to be done, *do* it, don't wait for somebody else to do it. And we'll think of each other as if we were all in the same family. We'll be a family. And we'll pray God to send us a whale." He bowed further and prayed in Iñupiat, then raised his head, and we got to our stations.

I was on a sled behind the second snowmobile. We went west along the beach, then down onto the ice. Here was a gap in the pressure ridge that ran along the shore, a gap already worn down by several snowmobiles. We entered and sped forward. I was seated on boards behind Annie and next to a double haunch of caribou, to whose roping I clung. The impact to my spine at each jolt was severe—we often fell ten inches suddenly, going at about thirty miles an hour. I grasped onto what I could to ease the shocks.

For the first time I was on the surface of the frozen ocean. From surface level it reminded me of the hedged fields of England, irregular like them and surrounded by tall barriers. Here the barriers consisted of upright and jostled ice blocks, pressure ridges caused by wind forcing huge ice sheets together. Between the barriers lay acres of smooth ice, faulted by shifts in their level and by intrusive earlier rifts, now frozen over and clear of snow. The snowmobile went over the lesser rifts unconcernedly, always making for convenient gaps in the barriers ahead, where previous crews with pickaxes had reduced the chaos in the gaps to some kind of track. Even so, the gaps were difficult hurdles, tests for the tough machines. Crossing one of them, we teetered upward, then fell disastrously into a puddle of water the other side. The snowmobile runners just bridged the pool, and we rushed on in a crazy curve and up onto a twelve-inch step of ice, taking it on one side only. A lurch. We did proceed, the snowmobile skids in front struggling with any obstacle ahead, propelled on inexorably by the tank-like caterpillar tracks behind, which ate into everything they encountered. The sled followed on its tether willy-nilly, rearing, side-shuffling, repeatedly falling, *smack*. I shifted the ruff up from my eyes to be able to foresee the bumps, anxious about life and limb.

After many "fields" we reached a wide parade of ice, much used by snowmobiles, with natural alcoves fifty feet wide at intervals. Here we could see tents occupying the alcoves. We were a mile and a half from the village as the crow flies and a mile and a half from the open water further out. We entered one of the empty alcoves and stopped.

Quickly, we unloaded the sleds and set up the tent. To anchor the guy ropes, we used a number of two-foot blocks of ice, cut out and dragged to the spot by the men. Plywood sheeting formed the floor of the tent, and immediately after the floor was laid, Gordon set the stove into place on the left, and Annie lit it, using driftwood and seal fat. I was the one to cut the seal fat. A dead seal, frozen solid, had been deposited outside to the right of the tent door. I was supposed to cut the fat into strips. It was tough tissue, that fat. Feeding the fire was an oddly emotional experience because of the sight of the dead body of the seal lying there and because of the running grease, the liquid-crisp sensation of cutting it with the curve of the ulu knife and forking up the tender piece with the stove fork, and the tricky conveyance of the strip past the door flap, into the tent, and into the dying stove, while I opened the door of the stove with the other hand. Would there be enough flame to avoid extinguishing the fire with that mass of cold energy? The thing to do was to place the strip delicately on burning driftwood sticks, where it would do the most good—then came the roar, the splutter, the great rewarding flame. It was a job that Annie also liked, for the same reason.

Gordon dragged a sled into the tent to make a bench on the right side and covered it with a caribou skin. His brother brought in the loaded grub box and put it by the left side wall beyond the stove, and Annie and I commenced to cook. The boy Sol brought us snow, and we melted it, cooked stew, made doughnuts, brewed coffee, loaded up our backpacks, and then took the meal to the men watching at the edge of the water. Later that day the ice started closing again, so we packed up the entire tent and returned to Ivakuk.

April 13, Wednesday.   Next day we were able to go down on the ice again, using the two snowmobiles. Sam went ahead to find a new campsite. As he rode on his machine, we could see his figure and face in serious consideration. His lips were pushed out in a wide pout. "Which is young ice? Which is old ice, suitable for a campsite and a tent with a stove?" We followed with our loaded sleds. We watched his stocky figure as his snowmobile veered this way and that; we watched his face already purpling with suntan. He had a big nose and deep cheeks. He was looking solemn because of his responsibilities, with his lower lip stuck out like that. I saw the graying hair under the hood and ruff, his practical brown hands, his head that could pray as well as think and plot. Sam Kasugaq.

The next campground was a mile from a wide expanse of water. After delivering food to the men by the water, I stayed with them and watched for a while. The scene was like an estuary: all was flat, wide, quiet, and sparkling. Through binoculars the distant waters in the sun's path appeared like millions of glittering crystals. Far away on the horizon was another ice bank with ice blocks that looked like palisades standing upright, owing to a trick of the light. A vague rectangle appeared to be suspended in mid air.

"See that? It's a polar bear," said Gordon.

A wide pool of water lay in front of us. The boat's stern was set on a block of ice so that the boat could be easily pushed into the water. Ice kept forming in the pool in front of the boat, so the young men started clearing the ice by throwing a line with a six-inch hook attached to it into the young ice, then pulling the line back and back to break a path through it. The men made channels on either side so that a large wedge of ice could be pushed out and broken up. However, the ice kept forming again. We ate some more of the stew; it was nearly cold. We swallowed another round of hot coffee and passed around the doughnuts. My warm clothes seemed to be doing a good job, and even my toes were toasty because they were encased in inner caribou socks made by Annie.

And I saw a whale.

This is what happened: one boat to the right of us started out after something and turned back; whatever it was lay about half a mile away. The distances were great. All was glitter, flatness, and the occasional sound of snowmobiles. Sam stood up. He heard the sound of blowing. Annie saw the whale first, in spite of her bad eye. "*Puiyaqpang-nguuq!* It's rising!" Sam took the binoculars, then handed them to me. There was the moving thing far away in the water—a long thing. As I watched, it moved like a curling mountain, with its big bow head, its taller and taller back—now it was mostly out of the water—huge—and then sank forward. It was too far away to chase, but the boat at the right tried for it, with the harpooner ready at the bow.

For weeks in town everyone had been making a forward rocking gesture with the hand. Now I knew what it meant.

April 14, Thursday.   Today a crisis occurred.

I was down on the ice beside the tent with Gordon and his sisters. Neither Sam nor Annie was with us. Gordon pointed out a large, fast-moving cloud, at first seen over us. Then more clouds appeared to emanate from a long, tube-shaped cloud over the southern cape. Gordon said quietly, "Put the food into the grub box; get those things put away." Then, "Pull those sleds out of the tent and load them." We were going to leave the ice and return to the village. Gordon and his brother took the tent down, and we loaded the sleds in short order. On the way up, passing the pressure ridges, twice I saw long, new cracks an inch wide. There didn't seem to be enough forces around to make those cracks—just a little wind. But some force made them.

Other forces were afoot. The whole town knew that the whale did not like film making. And they could see that the wind was turning south. The wind pushed all the ice together, shifted it, and jammed the open water shut. "The wind has gone south because the BBC man Nicholas Jones is in town," said Clem sadly, with a kind of bitter certainty. "The whales know, and they control the wind and the weather. They have senses that are much more than ours."

Clem began to speak deeply of the Iñupiat vision. "When things are right, our friendship covers all of us like a tent." I could see that. We wear our mammalian warm-blooded skins, and our parkas, and over us is the friendship that makes any environment possible and even fun. So it is not a matter of degrees of comfort: degrees of friendship override them by far.

That night I found it hard to write my notes, since I was so much involved. In addition to the fact that it was I who was hosting the BBC man in my house, I was afraid that my personal power, my Iñupiat generosity and "faith" as Clem called it, was not good enough. Nevertheless, my mind began to dwell on all the cultures that had the same kind of consciousness about their staple food: the Navajo with their revered sheep; the Athapaskans with the generous game; the Yaqui with the deer, a Christ-figure; Bangladesh with rice, holy rice; the Maya with corn, a deity for whose sake they lost the war with the Spaniards; the Japanese, for whom everything to do with the rice plant was sacred; the Christians with their bread and wine, which was Christ; the present-day Samaritans with their Passover lambs that went quietly to the sacrifice; the Africans with the antelope, their quarry—a visionary animal like the whale—which was the way it appeared when I saw the antelope in Africa. These comparisons balanced for me the strong local feeling in which I was caught up. It was a comfort that so many others found themselves carried along in the current of the same "food-piety." I was begging the whale to come.

The wind stayed south. Now Annie and Sam rarely talked about the whale, and when they did, they spoke quietly. Annie made another trip to her ice cellar and finished cleaning it. Then she felt better. She often went into the church to pray for a whale. An interval elapsed. The village was bored.

April 20, Wednesday. The Alaska Eskimo Whaling Commission representatives in Ivakuk finally refused permission to Nicholas Jones, the BBC man, to go down on the ice and film the whaling. He then left town; immediately the wind turned north at twenty-five miles per hour, and the water opened up again. The ice was now all different, with the water in a different position.

Clem told me later, "It was I who refused the BBC man. He'd have stopped the whales coming. The water wouldn't have opened. The minute he left, the water opened. Didn't it?" he demanded. "You call this superstition. I call it the truth."

"It's the truth," I said humbly.

The whale had much knowledge. It knew the condition of ice cellar and home; it would know if I turned children out of my house; it knew there was a movie man in my house; and it possessed the power to alter the weather. Clearly, the consciousness of the whale was getting to me.

April 23, Saturday. This time I walked down to the ice camp with little Gordon Junior, seven, who knew the way perfectly well along the shore and across the ice. It was good to find the tent and enter. The canvas spread above me. The sun showed through the weave because it was porous. I noticed small holes around the stovepipe exit and closed them with scotch tape. There was a smell of canvas in this space; the aroma of doughnuts; the scent of the snow and ice coming in from outside, fresh and stinging; the blast of the hot iron of the stove; the smell of the blood in the meat; the seductive and slightly repellent, fishy smell of seal; the smell of the various opened cans in front of the grub box—orangey Tang, cloying Crisco, coffee somewhere; the good smell of pilot crackers and flour—and then the unquestionably animal smell of the caribou skins covering the sled seats. It was invitingly comfortable; but work was facing me. I carried out the dish-washing water to a place forty feet out on the left and poured it down a sink hole in the ice that had already been formed by hot water slops. I made up the fire and cut up meat for the crew of thirteen who would appear at supper time. Annie turned up not long afterward to organize things and mix doughnuts.

After supper we played "Twenty-one," and I taught them "Cheating," a ridiculous card game in which you deliberately cheat your opponents, which I had learned from my brother Charlie. Louis, Luanne, and the tricky boy Sol cheated like mad.

"Very bad for the character," I said, deceptively putting down two cards at a time and winning. In the next game Louis sat on all his cards. Luanne announced the wrong number in such an authoritative voice that we never noticed. Trickiness proliferated like the wilderness of slabs around us. I howled with laughter at Louis's "innocent" face; it was my brother again, dark-haired, thinking, and tricky. Here in the present was another boy like him, laughing like the vile shamans do, a boy who had had shamanic experience himself. I was very happy. These young men were waiting to fight a whale; they were my sons all over again.

Life was heightened here on the ice, turned back and forth, a special experience with its own characteristic social odor, sweet, physical, and unmistakable, just as sex is. No one forgot that there existed that sea animal out there somewhere. The period of the whale hunt possessed an inevitability that ruled us. It was a liminal period, ancient and self-defined; it had the feel of a long-laid-down archetypal, physiological, even genetically endowed process, like childbirth or courtship: in this case, the process known as the approach of the hereditary hunter upon his catch. The whale was the hunter's host, both a sacramental host and a host in the social sense.

The young men with their playing cards, their cigarettes, and their soda pop—we were all enclosed in our tent, eyeing the luminous blue from the sunshine coming up from the gaps in the plywood floor, an unusual light from below, through ice. We were on a temporary floor. All was evanescent, as is a rite of passage. I wondered at the still yet unsteady unlikelihood of where we were. It is a major wonder of the universe why ice floats, why water becomes *lighter* when it becomes solid, not heavier. It has something to do with the clingability of electrons in the water molecule due to the peculiar character of hydrogen. I thank the funny universe. Otherwise, that day would have been nothing but a dream.

April 26, Tuesday, down by the water.   Gordon said, "Over there!" pointing to the west. He'd seen a boat enter the water after a whale and had seen the harpooner throw his weapon.

Before my eyes the crew were already sliding the boat into the water and were away, paddling west. I never followed what was done; it was so quick. There didn't seem to have been any splash when the boat entered the water. The thing was like a bird taking off, more integrated than a flock of birds—just one bird. Now it was here, now it wasn't. Very soon the boat was a tiny black silhouette against the dazzle path of the sun, and then it disappeared into the vast corridor of waters. The women left behind could see it turn toward a bay where Matthew's boat was floating. I could not see a thing for dazzle. We heard later that five boats gathered there in quick time, but there was nothing for them to pull in. Matthew's bomb had failed to explode. The result was one point less on the quota. Ivakuk now had only four strikes remaining out of the five.

Annie was miserable. "That Estelle!" she said, referring to Matthew's wife. "She talks funny to me." Annie screwed up her eyes. No one should talk funny during whaling. The wife should pray and be generous and calm. Matthew's name was mud.

But there was still watching to do.

15

The Whale's Head

Presence and Absence

May 1, Sunday. Annie and I were walking over the ice. We came to one of the many faults, a slight change of level in the frozen sea. We both stopped for a moment to take off our parkas because it was hot. Annie suddenly stood erect. Her hand went out. "Ta! Ta! . . . They've caught a whale. . . . Clem's caught a whale." Her hand flashed to her midriff. "And we will have the stomach share." How did she know that?

"Yes. The Jacksons." she said, and began to dance about and laugh with pleasure. She flung her arms around my neck. Hardly awake to the situation, I began to laugh.

It was indeed the case, as we found out from our tent neighbors who had a CB walkie-talkie. Clem had caught a whale, and our crew was the second boat to arrive on the scene. Thus, we were all going to receive "second boat" shares.

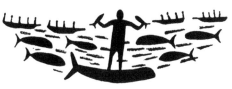

Many times after that day Annie described to her friends the scene by the ice fault, and especially the certainty that came to her that we would get the stomach share. Her hand would always flash to her midriff. "Didn't I say so, Edie?" And she would laugh.

This was a signaling in of Clem's whale, in the same way that the first whale caught by Annie's own crew was sighted and signaled in by Annie herself. It was on her birthday, as she often told me. On the occasion of Clem's present whale, that original gesture of Annie's, out on the ice, itself constituted the knowledge that we would have the stomach share. The gesture *was* the knowledge. She felt the shares "in her stomach." It was a gesture given to her by some sort of communication with the whale. There had been many crews out. It did not have to be Clem's whale, and we did not have to come in second. The woman's connection with the whale was shown in this episode as a state of attunement.

We heard the close-up account of the catching of Clem's whale in fragments afterward. Clem had never caught a whale before. His boat was old, his snowmobile was almost defunct, and he had only his brother's three-wheeler Honda to rely on. His standing among Westernized Iñupiat in the village was in question because he was a Iñupiaq patriot, strong for the renewal of his culture.[1]

At the time of the event, Clem had been down on the edge of the ice beside an inward curve of the water, asleep on a caribou-covered sled after a bout of watching. And lo, a whale rose exactly in front of him. Hearing the spout, Clem awoke. The great body was revealed in plain sight. He seized his harpoon. It was told that he trembled—he trembled as he raised the harpoon with both hands—and he flung. *Boom!* It happened. The whale was his, but it was precisely not his; because it was his first whale, he was bound to give it entirely away. Meanwhile, there was the work of cooperation among the helping boats to administer further blows and to tow the beast in.

Catching the whale was in a sense Clem's accolade. The village thereafter began to recognize Clem's worth and value his traditionalism.[2]

But what of Margie, the wife of Clem, the whaling captain? Margie told me that some time before, at the full moon before whaling started, she and Netta and Clem's sister-in-law had gone out into the moonlight, taking a bowl of water, just as Annie described. Margie raised the bowl to the moon and prayed for food for the children and for Clem to catch a whale. "You have to pray aloud," she said when recounting the event.

"In Iñupiat?" I asked.

"You can use your own words," she said. "And look, we go catch a whale!" A White man staying in the village openly termed this "magical thinking." Clem knew that White people called it magic, and as usual he taxed me with it. I said patiently, "No, it's not magic, it's real."

"Too many things have happened together," said Margie. "When the BBC man left town, we began to catch whales.³ And you know how the whaling captain's wife has to walk slow? I was walking slow the very time Clem caught the whale. Aaka 'grandmother' was around. She said to me, 'Margie, why are you walking so slow?' It was she herself who always told me to walk slow or the whale wouldn't come. And at that very moment Clem was catching the whale. Afterward I asked Clem, 'When you struck it, did it go away quickly?' 'No, it went *slowly*.' You see, slow. I was in the laundromat carrying the bags in, and I wanted to hurry, I was—like—half hurrying and half slow, and I made myself slow.⁴ I tell you Edie, I was crying after they told me he'd caught a whale. I didn't believe them. Also there were so many things I'd have to do, and I didn't know half of them." Margie was a Yup'ik Eskimo, not from a whaling culture. "Aaka was home. We were very happy, and lots of people were there."

We heard that Clem's men had cut off the tail flippers of the whale and sent them to Margie. The wife is always given the flippers. Margie and the women saw to it that the huge pieces were put in her ice cellar for the Whaling Festival. ∎

Not long after, Marlene and I set off to the scene of Clem's whale. We could see from afar silhouetted figures, then a tent, which we passed, then a group assembled by the water. I went along a little and looked into the water. A black thing lay mostly submerged, with black, rubbery objects tied around it with ropes. These were the arm flippers tied together. The tail flippers had already been cut off, and some muktuk cut off from the flank was already being boiled in a large pan in the tent. Sam had been served some boiled muktuk and was eating it hungrily. He told me later that he got a "stomach" from it, diarrhea, because it was still too fresh.

The task of hauling in the whale was yet to come. No tractors would be used, for this was not a commercial enterprise. Tackle arrived from the village, summoned by CB radio: huge cables, pulley blocks, and a webbing wrap to go around the tail. The men proceeded to dig two separate pairs of holes in a flat area of ice, some way back from the water. The holes went down thirty inches or so and reached the sea water. A hawser was led underneath through the water from one adjacent hole to another, by means of a hook on the end of a long pole; then each end of the hawser was joined on top of the ice into a loop, so that the intervening ice acted as a stanchion for the main hauling rope. The second pair of holes had the same function, but this time the stanchion was installed to anchor the continuation of the rope after it passed through the tail collar wrap of the whale and back to the pulley block system, so that when we hauled on the main rope that was passed through the final end of the block system, we were pulling in the whale in low gear. Such a tackle was needed because the whale weighed over forty tons, and hauling it in was always tricky, with slippage and delays.[5]

The entire crowd manned the rope. As I hauled, my woolen gloves on the rope grew soaked with melt water, but my hands were warm at all times. The wool of the gloves was soon in tatters. I had to haul walking backward, eyeing behind me for what we were backing up to, such as small pressure ridges, cracks, pools, and slippery places. But we continued. Clem shouted, "Aaa-ll the way! Aaa-ll the way!" as we dug in at each major tug. I came to know every bit of that ice as we progressed backward, then repeatedly came forward to take up the slack every time they shortened the pulley system. I came to know each drop and jag and fault and fragment of ice. I put my all into it, as everybody else did, and felt the tiny arthritis ache in my right hip again. It was eased by a rest and some tea and donuts, served beside the windbreak. We returned to the rope and hauled again, seeing at the edge of the water in front of us a huge object gradually appearing, upside down. It was almost there. Its vast form now dominated the scene.

"Go up and look," said Sam. I approached close. The first thing I saw, along the side of the tilted body, was the exposed ventral slit, delicately fringed around with hair at the navel. Through the lower end of this slit, as if it were the undercarriage of a plane, appeared the penis, three feet long, curvy, white, and somehow very attractive. The ordinary skin itself is its foreskin, the member appearing through it when the call comes. Death, as in most mammals, including male humans, was one such a call. The anus showed, small and delicately tufted. It was a beautiful whale that had come to us, now mostly dead except for the spirit, which was immortal, in the head.

I looked at the head, stationed with its chin to the top now and its eyes downward. The chin bore striking patterns of white and black, the animal's only marking. Already one could see some baleen protruding from its mouth (baleen are those vast vertical shutters, black in color, that sift the whale's food). Hair grew wildly around and between the vanes; this hair helps the sifting. The animal must have experienced hair in his mouth like an old man drinking his tea through his mustache. When the men started the cutting, I was able to see the tongue, a six-foot monument of pinkish gray and white marbled flesh, set plentifully with black taste buds inches across, resting now on the upturned roof of the mouth, which also bore a ferocious pattern of black taste buds among the fat. The tongue was beautiful in its curve, like a modern sculpture. That tongue could never talk as we can, for not enough of it was free of the mouth; in fact, only a few inches projected from the base. But it was an immense organ of compression and decompression, drawing in and expelling the water continually for the sifting and swallowing of krill and plankton. And it could also sing.

There was the sound of a snowmobile. Everyone looked back. "It's Margie. Margie's here." She dismounted and strode straight to her whale, to where Clem stood beside it. They joined in a great hug—husband and wife. All those years had been hard on Clem and Margie. Now they had made it. My eyes were wet. Where was my Vic?

There was work to do in the Jackson family. The dismemberment of the whale had to be performed with care. This would be better termed *dismantling* because the flesh and the body, apart from its head, were its mantle, its "parka," as they called it. The first cuts were made by the small and stubby village preacher. With face intent, he scored with his knife-tipped pole two straight lines a foot apart right down the whale's side, at the "belt." There was no arguing about shares. Indulging in conflict would repel all whales and close the ice. The correct pattern of meat division was in every schoolchild's exercise book: the captain's share, first boat, second boat, third boat, right to the eighth boat.

The dismantling process was performed with the correct tools: the long-handled knife, the square-ended joint severer, stout hooks on long poles, and short knives. No axes or saws were used. This was no time to break bones; the bones would be separated as whole pieces. I looked carefully at the process. Each cut was first made with a little action of probing. There was not a single emotional act while they were cutting. As they carved into the white mass, the cutting of the fat sounded like cutting crisp, solid sugar: *slutch, slutch, slutch;* meanwhile, six men hauled on a hook set in the adjacent flesh to assist the cutting. They were easing out a large three-foot-by-one-foot-by-one-foot slab of skin and fat. They tugged until at last a separation occurred—with a thud and a splash onto the puddled ice. Then, laughing, they grasped the block of fat by the rope attached to the hook, turned, and all of them marched off, dragging the block after them at a run, keeping in step, toward their correct place in the array of shares that was already spreading out on the ice. Each boat crew was in charge of cutting and hauling its own share, so these laughing bands were brothers, cousins, or bilateral in-laws.

In the course of time they managed to cut off the tail entirely, then dug into the belly and released a mighty waterfall of warm blood, which soaked the ice for thirty feet around. It was the first river sound I had heard since the previous August. After that, little streamlets of blood kept pouring out. One spout fountained for some time. The smell was desirable, foody, and a little maddening. There was another strange sound, a gurgle from the stomach that elicited a cry of wonder from all. That cry from the people was the one voice of emotion, the underground emotion in which everyone was bathed.

The sight of the red and black and white mound being continually divested stays in my memory. The guts were hanging out at one side. The ribs and sternum were already taken off and were standing on one side like a great red boat. Men were occupied with digging into a rib where it was attached to the sternum, using the square-ended joint severer, striking and striking into the tough gristle that linked and cushioned the bones. Meanwhile, two men with hooks hauled at the sections upon which the cutters were working in order to widen the gap and make the hacking easier. The men all had wet feet from the puddles made by the heat of the whale's body. And so it would go on for twenty-four hours. Incessantly they labored to disrobe the leviathan of its fifteen-inch-thick muktuk parka: now they were hacking very knowledgeably at the disk joints of the vertebral column. They took out the arms from their shiny cup joints and laid the arms upon the ice like the sides of buildings, leaving the ball of the joint protruding, shiny and smooth, harder than ordinary bone. I felt it. It was like opaque marble, perfect.

The lungs, kidneys, liver, and stomach still lay attached in a terrific homogeneous gray mass, slobbery and slack, ten feet across. The stomach had been ruined by the gunpowder of the bomb. The men meanwhile cut off the black muscle meat in ragged masses and dragged them to the meat division areas. They eased off after this point. The red mound, the body of the whale, had gone. The division sets were to be seen in a wide circle around the carcass, with blood tracks going to each one—a scene of white ice, orange-red tracks, sunshine, and startling black and white muktuk blocks laid out in thoughtful order. The bluish-black skin, ribbed like fingerprints and tasting extremely good, was a different black from the nearly black blood meat.

The work had been proceeding with a forward momentum, with continuous energy, moved by the spirit of hunger, hunger for food of great value that was theirs for the digging. A film crew would have spoiled the quiet happiness, the "us-ness" that reigned. Clem showed me the ear of the whale, with its six-inch tympanum, the ear drum, on one side of it, soft and sensitive like an inverted baby's cheek, and on its other side showing a hard polished conch with a curved echo chamber. He wanted me to see it because this is what had been listening to us. Clem's manner was quiet, his face a combination of smile and deadpan.

At last it was midnight, but we could still see. The immense single bone arch of the lower jaw still reared out of the skull. All was upside-down, the position in which the whale had died. The skull was now visible as an enormous red three-chambered edifice twelve feet across, mounted in front with the great jawbone. All this had to wait. Standing in the gloom of twilight, I heard Vera and Madeline say, "Margie must take out the heart. It's Margie. The woman." My ears pricked up. What I was hearing referred to the wife's identification with the body of the whale—with in fact its very heart. I saw six women help Margie do the cutting, and eventually the heart, two feet across, lay separated on the ice. It was the women who cut up the organs, heart, kidneys, and intestines, and I worked alongside, packing curiously honeycombed kidney slabs into sacks and loading them onto the waiting snowmobiles, the lights of which now looked dazzling and lighted up the women as they continued to labor on the dim floor of bloody ice.

"You should use gunny sacks," said Vera. "Yes," said Margie. "These big plastic bags aren't strong enough."

"Don't forget to keep the meat ten days in the cold store before you start fermenting it," advised Vera. The women intended to make *mikigaq* "fermented blood meat," a delicacy for the whaling festival. The maturing process had to be carefully controlled to obtain the best flavor.

At last in the newly growing light of morning we left and took our loads home.

Thinking back over the impact the whale made on me, I remember my first glimpse of the black mound reared high over the ice. Going near, I felt its overshadowing presence, with its life closed down, the eye low on the side, matte and dark, the machinery of baleen all silent like organ pipes without wind. This whale was a hill. Its tail flippers were amputated, and there was even a section already cut from the side. "Pierced feet and side?" Yes, it was the Pietà scene on the lap of mother ice. Then the work, the driving performance with knives and hacking irons and the cooperating rhythm of men leaning on ropes, setting their feet in unison, pulling. The black figures were sometimes seen against dazzling ice, sometimes against the blue of the sea, constantly changing position and re-forming upon another section of the beast, methodically heaving off its immense parka, then dragging each section to its designated owner, and working on the spine—a different task, needing skill to get inside the complexity of the tail and spine joints. Removing the baleen was a very difficult job because the hardest tissue apart from bone was the roof of the mouth and lip. The cold wind and sun were always about us, the sound of splashing of feet, the occasional heavy thud of falling segments, the odor of nourishing blood—a reassuring odor; the quietness and warm joy of the men, shown in their willingness, plainly shown in body language, though rarely in their faces. Most of the time I was sitting on a block of ice, watching. Clem's son Kehuq noticed something in the carcass, went forward, and drew out part of a brass metal tube. It was the bomb.

Annie said, "Poor whale. Poor whale. They feel." I knew they did, self-sacrificial souls, coming toward their human brothers to suffer for their sake. "We the whales do what we must and suffer because of our unity with you. Then there will be a greater good."

The last panels of skin and fat came away. The nearer muktuk was hauled free with much pulling this way and that. All was laid in order. The huge jawbone, fifteen feet long, still rose from the head like a phallus. I saw that the head was much wider than it was spherical because of the two massive projecting bone processes extending to the eyes on each side. Walking around the mass, I located the nerve endings of the eyes, mere stumps; and between the wide projections, exactly in the middle of the brain case, I saw the hacked-off spinal cord, the nerve cord of the body. All the rest of the nerve world was enclosed in a four-foot-wide bloody lump hiding the complicated bone of the skull. The skull lump was set between those side wings that guarded the eyes, all overtopped by the rearing arch of the jawbone. Inside the skull—what? No one would look. "We never eat that," said Annie. Inside it—? I stood facing it as before a wall, wondering. ▪

May 2, Monday.   Next morning I came back to the ice. The head was still there, the only thing remaining on the ice. Clem and his men were standing around it. He had already told me that the spirit of the whale was alive inside it, and if the head were released into the water the spirit would be able to grow its parka again and return.

The men drew away for a moment. Clem prepared them for the last task, the giving of the head to the sea, the work of *niaquq*. For the last time they tied ropes onto the jawbone, and Ernie stationed them along the ice margin beyond the head. They pulled, with a wrenching tug. They came to this side, others steadying the head behind. They wrenched on the rope, rocked, attempting to rear the solid skull mass out of the pit in the ice that its own heat had melted. They wrenched and at last the head was free of the hole, standing on ice nearer the edge. Now it was a matter of going back to the sea rim on the far side and pulling, then forward to the rim on the near side and pulling, edging the head crabwise toward—toward that drop-off into the deep ocean. It took half an hour. Steadily they pulled, exchanged sides, pulled, and the head crept toward the edge. When it was at the edge itself they detached the ropes and all got behind the skull and pushed, straining with all their might, their gloves wringing with blood. Heave! It moved. Heave! It moved. It teetered. Heave. SPLASH.

Suddenly Vic was in my mind. The nobility of the animal, the Viking funeral, the crew doing the last honors. My face was streaming, and Clem glanced at me.

Instantly drawing into a line, they howled, "Ui-ui-ui! Yuuuuu!" and rocked with joy. The spirit, iñua, was returned. All around there was a sigh of relief, for the ice was clear of it, its red shadow released into the dim water. Everything was quite all right now. All that was left on the ice were the men and their shares—material things, ordinary. That great spirit presence was gone. Without the head the stretches of ice looked quite different, a vacant lot. So a spirit had been there. And as the yells died down one more shout arose, "Come back!"

Now I remembered what the whale wanted, the greater good. When the head was back in the water, we did know the whale's spirit, we did become conscious of it, which was the whale's purpose in coming to us. Absence equals presence. Consciousness of absence proves former presence. Some would call this no proof, but it happened. My knowledge did deepen. The whale did come, it was somehow in tune with us and we with it. The events were those kinds of events, they had that shape, not any other.

And now our whale had gone to grow its new parka, to reincarnate, "reflesh" itself, and join the cosmic cycle that rolls forward in continuous replenishment. The whale as a conscious being had grown to be the dominant experience of all the ocean-dwelling Iñupiat.[6]

The anthropology of hunting is no easy matter. It might be said that the anthropology of hunting would be impossible if the object were to systematize. For an ethnographer participating in hunting, the *play* of events is the material, and hunting as a manner of acting will produce "flashes" in the writing, like the flashes produced in the process of hunting animals. In Ivakuk the flashes in actual hunting were what the people expected and understood, and the flashes themselves originated in the *random*. Basically, the arrival of a particular whale was a random event, from the perspective of the world of cause and effect. The randomness affecting a hunter like Clem therefore keyed him into a different world from ours—different in time, too, since the random play of events in a hunter's life created "hunting time," especially during whaling, which even the strictness of high school hours could not subvert. (That year the Iñupiat school board at last decided to allocate a maximum total of ten days subsistence leave for hunter youths, allowable whenever the whale appeared.) Randomness was expected; it was the norm for the hunters' world. This did not foster some form of unenlightened magical thinking, the imputation of which so concerned Clem, but out of this rare kind of environment arose something real. Clem knew that the spirits of the ancient masters and of the whale were able to operate in that world and were able to substantiate principles such as "the whale will come if you pray to the moon," or "the whale opens the water." This kind of knowledge allowed a hunter like Clem to retain shamanic power. His center could live "out there," in that liminal space, and make connections with the animals. Clem's success spun on something like the divining spinning top that was used to link the people into the future seasons, and he wanted it like that, wanted the fit to be loose enough to accommodate spirit intervention. The craze for bingo, the gamble, was a modern substitute for this environment of the random. The hunters were quiet men, not only because they had become accustomed not to disturb the game they were stalking, but also because their random world reached down into their very souls. I use the term *soul* advisedly. There is an invisibility of the soul itself, like the existence of a shard of glass in a glass of water. There was no cozy domesticity in these men, nor could there be. They were forever hanging loose. The great whaling captain Ezra Lowe's last wish, so he told me before he died of cancer, was to go upriver to his caribou hunting grounds on the tundra.

Through the flow of activity in a random environment, this May, the whale spirit was able to come into focus. Alongside, parallel with the activities of whaling, was the narration of the hunt, its second life. The narrations vitalized and sharpened perception, just as Margie's account of the laundromat, told after the event, sharpened it for her, and so did Annie's story of the stomach share, for her. Perception was focused for everybody as the stories were told. In the same way my own accounts, describing personal experience for the most part, and the way they were because of the person I was—not able to imitate the Iñupiat style, of course—were for me a way to my own sharpened perception. ∎

16
Rich Parkas and Festival Food

May 7, Saturday. At this time all the elders of the village were being presented with portions of muktuk by the hunters of the five whales that were eventually caught, the last two simultaneously. The freezer of my refrigerator was full, and I was proud. Marlene and I were also learning to discriminate between good muktuk and bad.

Now we heard the whale hunt stories; the village was full of jokes and storytelling. I happened to see Janet in the senior van. Janet was an *umialik* "whaling captain," a widow running the boat of her son Don, who was the harpooner, and Don had caught a whale. Janet told us how she and her sister, who was from outside, had climbed up on a pressure ridge to watch—when suddenly the whale surfaced. The men launched the boat, but Janet could not see what was happening because of her bad eyesight. Her sister, standing beside her on the ridge, gave a running commentary on the drama going on down in the water, so that Janet would know what was happening—how the boat approached the whale and how Don lifted up his harpoon to strike. Janet told us that her sister at her side not only described the scene but actually copied Don's gestures, adding the live action to the verbal commentary. Now as we went along in the senior van, Janet copied the actions for us. Don struck the whale. Janet saw the sister's arms plunge, "striking the whale." In the senior van Janet's arms plunged.

Now, back in the verbal story, Janet said, "My sister and I suddenly heard the bomb go off. My sister fell flat on her face"—we all laughed—"right there on the ice. She just lay there with her hands over her eyes." By this time the senior van, as on many previous occasions, was in pandemonium.

"A minute went by. 'Can I come up now?' said the sister." (We were back on the ice. The sister imagined something like a megaton bomb had gone off, with fragments all over the place.) Janet herself was in fits, telling the story to the elders as the senior van swayed about on its route through the village.

[Iñupiat people revel in building a story that includes various levels of reported speech, just as they revel in their varied and extended sense of spirit things. The added touch of the sister's miming, coupled with the sister's genuine terror—and all at second hand—constituted a tour de force that was the Iñupiat story connoisseur's delight. Now I am telling the story of the story of the story in my own way.]

Janet told me she had had a great deal of help with the cutting of the whale, cooking, and so on. "I've done nothing," she said.

Another story: Annie happened to be visiting in my house while I was telling Marlene about a novel of Doris Lessing's I was reading, about squatters in a house who did not take care of it but stored buckets of feces on the top floor. Annie got interested and said suddenly, "Make mikigaq of 'em." We went into gales of laughter, as the joke was horribly apt. Many women in the village were fermenting whale meat in barrels, in preparation for the approaching whale festival.

The whale in all its spirituality comes to us to be our food; we sour its meat as a finger-licking delicacy, then make jokes like that about it. I was giddy with these swings of mood.

May 14, Saturday. Annie told me how, one day, when Sam was a little boy, he and his dad had gone to the cemetery. "That big cross, you remember that big cross?" Annie stretched her arm up high. "Sam saw—on top of the cross—" she lowered her voice—"*Something!* 'Dad, can you see that thing on top of the cross; it's white, up there on top?' 'No, there's nothing there, son.' His dad couldn't see it. What was it? Sam watched it and it flew up and went away. Was it an angel? Maybe it was his imagination. He was only a little boy."

Annie was asking *me*. I was often asked this kind of thing, for instance when Claire asked me what I thought when she told me that she once saw human footprints turn into those of a bear, and when Stella asked me if the ice really widened when the woman shaman sang over a crack. Five different people at the whale hauling asked me what I thought about the whaling, and I answered it was an excellent thing, and that the International Whaling Commission should scrap the quota system for subsistence people and let the Iñupiat do what they had done for centuries, take as many whales as they needed. There was a hint that my questioners thought that my being English would mean that I was in favor of Greenpeace and would be against the whaling. For my part I was trying to figure out how the Iñupiat viewed the Americans and other outsiders such as myself. I could see how Clem felt about my puzzling presence in the village. I could see his bitter experience speaking during our talks on shamanism. He himself never asked me questions but went right ahead and accused me of disbelief and positivism. He was aggressive, and in my opinion, in general, he had a right to be.[1] ∎

Answering Annie was not hard. I knew of many miracles of angels. It was no good saying it was just Sam's imagination. That argument fails to get a grip on real events that happen to be strange. "If he saw it, it wasn't his imagination." I said. "He saw it, and he remembers it. It could have been an angel," I said.

Annie went on, "Ever since then, Sam knew he had to do things for people. He became store manager, mayor of Ivakuk, head of the Ivakuk Native Corporation, he was high on the regional corporation board, and he was the local head of the Alaska Eskimo Whaling Commission. He had cancer"—and Annie gave a dramatic account of his hospital cure. Another fact that emerged was that Sam's last name used to be Jackson. He was actually a relative of Clem's. But he changed his name to Kasugaq because, it was said, he wanted to have an Iñupiat name.

May 21, Saturday.   The snow finally melted. Far out to the east, by Traderstown, along the beach toward the mountains, little purple flowers were blooming, tiny pads with a lip of minute flowers on the south side of each. The grass was just beginning to show among last year's dry stalks. Marlene and I found a huge whale jawbone frozen into the soil. Blue pools appeared among the massed ice fragments on the sea. There seemed to be no mess or slush at the time of thaw, just quiet beauty. On land, on the tundra toward the lagoon, we saw open water like gashes of royal blue—a deeply emotional sight—with geese from above descending and settling. There was a pair at the far side of the brilliant water, which was so blue it was dark. The birds were quietly floating. Sandpipers flew in pairs low to the ground. A flock of small brown sea gulls were simply standing about, and they never flew off as we walked by them. Fine brown sand appeared further on, and driftwood; over on the right the ice fields of the sea itself were topped with a line of blue-black on the horizon, canopied by a light vapor, the water cloud. Squirrels—*sikrit* is the only word for them—stood up on an old sod house mound like small people and looked at us fixedly. They said *"Tit-tit-tit,"* then flirted their black and orange tails twice like flag signals and jumped head first into their holes. Looking up, I saw the land stretched before me in a bewildering mirage as far as the mountains. And then the mountains took over the horizon, extending across a quarter of the entire rim of the earth in white and blue peaks and dips, along toward the sea, merging at last into the haze of the southern cape. The sun was high, like a spring noon in England.

We returned at length, past defunct camps, to the village, which was just the same as ever with its hard streets, children on Honda three-wheelers, and the houses. It was ordinary home.

May 24, Tuesday. Visiting at Netta's, I plucked up courage and told her that I had been making spirit trips, trying to develop the Native-American ability. As usual when I referred to matters of my personal spirit, she made no direct comment, but responded with something from her own experience.

She began to talk of the childhood illness she had mentioned before on September 17, enacting it in dialogue in her skilled way and giving it much detail. "I was only eight," she said. "I was very thin—very thin. You know I was dying." Her eyes rounded. "I *ku-tuck*ed all the time; I fell over and couldn't walk. I couldn't eat." Poor little kid.

"My father's sister came to treat me." This was her Aunt Judy, who was a shaman. "She had prepared a small bit of whale meat—just a little bit, don't you know"—and Netta squeezed up two fingers. "I wouldn't eat it.

"'I don't like it.'" Netta screwed up her mouth pitifully.

"'You have to eat it, *or you will die.*'

"At last I took it in my mouth. And I managed to swallow it. Now Aunt Judy sang to the whale meat—she spoke to it in my stomach." Netta pointed to her stomach.

"'Come up! Bring that bad thing up!' You see, a shaman put a bad thing in there. 'Come out!'

"Aunt Judy called to it to work its way out through my abdomen. She called and waited. The bad thing came up and up, by the power of that whale meat, up into the skin of my abdomen—and out! Aunt Judy had her hands like this"—Netta cupped her hands—"on my stomach. The bad thing came out, and she caught it in her hands. She took it along carefully and blew it out up the smoke hole."[2]

"Then I went to sleep," Netta went on wonderingly. "I never could sleep before. I slept without waking. My mother kept trying to wake me in case I was dead. At last after a whole day I awoke. I was feeling light, light! I was hungry. They gave me food, and I recovered."

Netta repeated a number of instances of shamanism used by her or others of her family. I did not need to fear that shamanism was disappearing, nor did I need to feel ashamed of confessing my own low-grade form of shamanism. Whenever I mentioned such things, the telling precipitated many narratives.

Preparing for the Whaling Festival. **May 30, Monday.**   In June the village was going to celebrate its five whales at the traditional Whaling Festival. At Netta's I saw Margie stitching a festival parka for her step-daughter, and beside it lay a new parka already cut out for old Auntie Nora, the tiny adopted daughter of Netta. Margie's sister was having her parka made from black velveteen. Clem's captain-style parka, in peacock blue, was waiting to have its trimmings completed. Margie had been up since 5:00 A.M. because it was only two weeks until the Whaling Festival.

May 31, Tuesday.   Annie's mikigaq was ready. She sent for us to taste it. I put my hand in the barrel and pulled from the mass a ragged scrap of fermented whale meat swimming in black juice. It sparkled like champagne; it was fizzy. When I chewed it I could taste a delicate, sweet dryness, what we call brut, while at the same time it was very juicy. The stuff was absolutely black, with just the right tenderness. It was better than caviar. Each woman-captain was concerned about the fermentation just now and was taking much care about it.

The same was true for the making of new parkas. These were the subject of much discussion and gossip among the active women of the village. The application of fancy trimmings was a carefully considered business. The trimmings were all different. Some women took two different-colored lengths of rickrack and twisted them cunningly together in neat zigzags, then stitched them onto the bottom of the coat in curled and looped arabesques interspersed with regularly arranged whorls, loops, or patterns in yet another color. The impact was startling and glorious. Others followed the traditional method of sewing on five or seven bands of bias binding in a single color that contrasted with the coat color, then interleaving little echelons, diamonds, and chevrons made of squares of bias binding in a variety of colors.

In all cases the parka was supposed to show wolverine or beaver peeking out from below the hem, as if the whole coat were lined with it inside. The dressmaker sewed the wolverine strip at the hem in alternating sections of light and dark fur to create a wave effect. She would have to spread the parka on the floor, then get down and lay out different pieces of wolverine around the hem to try them out, with some sighing and retrying [just as in writing this book I had to lay out the pieces first and try them out, sighing, but proudly feminine in this kind of work]. Her tiny sharp ulu knife was ready to trim each piece of fur to the right size. Then she would "skin-sew" the pieces together in a long strip, and finally sew the strip on. Meanwhile, two or three babies would be trying to get at the scissors.

The ruff also received detailed attention. Often it was made with soft wolf fur around the neck and then radiated out in wolverine, finally ending in an enormous halo with scalloped wolf tips at intervals all around the circumference. My own ruff was wolverine only, which prickled slightly but was a great boon because I could close it up almost completely over my face in the subzero wind chills and still breathe, and never be afraid of being iced up.

For the coming festival Annie made me a new parka with a polar bear ruff plus flower trimmings at the hem. Many times when I was going along the street, some friendly woman would come up and admire my new parka. "Who made it?"

"Annie." And the woman would pick up the hem to check on the stitching inside. Each of them had a professional eye for good stitching.

June 2, Thursday. When I was in the school office today to do some photocopying, there was a power failure. Robert Nashanik, who was employed as janitor, was in the office at the same time, as well as the school undersecretary, who was the wife of the Assembly of God elder. We had to wait in the inner gloom for the light to go on and the computers to begin again. Robert was in conversation with the secretary.

"Do you know what happened to me? Listen to this; it'll show you what I've been talking about. I and my friend Greg were down on the ice hunting. Greg was with the snowmobile in one place, and I was in another. The ice seemed thick enough." Robert put his hands one over the other, five inches apart. "But a lot of it was thin. Then I met a polar bear." Robert's eyes widened. "There it was standing up at me. I leveled my gun and shot it. It was a glancing blow. You could see the red coming out on the fur of its leg." Robert put his hand on his own leg. "About there." I stiffened as I pictured this. A dangerous situation.

"I got back from that bear pretty quick and tried another shot. There was something wrong with the gun, and it wouldn't fire. I wrestled with the gun. Nothing worked." We two women gasped. Robert sat there, so he must have escaped.

"The ice was flat all around for miles. I didn't look for the snowmobile or anything, not even my gun. I just ran. I ran half a mile *very quickly*." Robert grinned. "Then I stopped. Where was Greg? I couldn't see him anywhere on that flat ice. I saw an tall pressure ridge in the distance and went to it and climbed to the top. From there I saw a black dot far away, and I went toward it. It was Greg. He was *swimming*." We gasped again. Robert went on, "Greg had driven onto thin ice in the snowmobile and had fallen in, and he couldn't get out of the water. He was just there swimming. I ran toward him, but of course I found the ice was thin.

"I called to him, 'Break off the ice; break it off where you can, and I'll be able to get to you.' He broke it off. I had with me only a short piece of rope, you know, real short." He showed us the length with his arms, about five feet.

"I lay down on the ice"—and Robert bent forward a little with his arm out—"with my rope. What could I do? The rope was so short. I prayed and threw it to him. It stretched," said Robert softly, looking puzzled. "Like elastic. It became long. Greg took the end and I pulled him out. It was hard to do because he was wearing a jacket with a lambskin lining, and it was soaked and very heavy. He still had his gun looped around his body. So he never lost his gun."

Now the lights came on, and we went about our business.

Here, Robert, like the others, didn't seem to claim strange powers for himself; he was just surprised at how things happened. The stereotype of the egotistic, triumphant shaman was rare except in cases of jealousy. Then, evilly intended deeds were just as likely to turn against the sorcerer.

So it would not do for me to praise Robert's abilities. His character had been shown in his previous deeds.

June 3, Friday. Going up Margie's steps, I smelled the fragrance of champagne. Inside her porch I found three women bent over wooden barrels of mikigaq with their arms up to their elbows in the dark red blood, turning over the meat in order to keep the fermenting process good and even, without pockets of air. Margie was one of the women. Her arms were thin. "It's hard work," she gasped, stretching her back for a bit.

"It smells just fine," I said.

Later on, Marlene and I visited Annie and found her on the floor of the living room in the midst of a huge mass of tangled dressmaking trimmings that she was trying to sort out. Marlene and I got down to the job of untangling them. There was rickrack all of gold; lengths of silver sequins; strings of multicolored fret designs in green, red, and gold; multicolored green, gold, blue, and silver bar designs; rows of woolly pink and green flowers; yellow woolly stars hanging from a bar; rivers of one-color red, green, and white rickrack—all of them zigzagging and coiling in the frenzied tangle. We drew out the prettiest first and rolled them up, leaving the brown and black ones until the end. Meanwhile, Annie got busy on the sewing machine.

June 5, Sunday. Some of my photographs arrived back from the processors in Seattle. I showed them to various people who happened to come by. Some of the photos were pictures of last year's fall events, and some showed winter scenes.

Looking at the photographs, I was reminded again of the darkening fall, the withered grasses, the gray slush ice forming on the ocean, and the scouring snows of midwinter, especially the curious marks of drifts seen around the houses. And there in one photo was Annie's house with a fringe of sunset behind it. I had taken that one at noon on December 21. I remembered the secret lowering development of ice through the dark months, the grind heard at nights beyond the wind, presaging the manufacture of what everyone was looking forward to in March, the revelation of the GREAT ICE all the way to the horizon. I remembered first seeing the vast "fields and hedges" out at the point when trying to fish with Annie. This was the stage, the boards on which the drama was to be played, the scene of the primal act of the people, a stage ready and prepared for the action to begin—a stage prowled by polar bears, for it was their domain.

In the new sunlight in March, the human population gathered itself together and likewise prepared its complex equipment. This was a population knowledgeable and adept in the prediction of what had not yet happened. It prepared itself for the second revelation from behind that ice stage—WATER, the open lead. Within and up between the ice, which was the first "stage," there appeared water, which was like another curtain opening behind. First, then, came the transition from darkness to light and the preparation of the stage that was the ice; second, from the stage itself to its inverse and opposite, water. There had to be boats and the step-by-step getting into gear of the whaling technology and equipment. And I remembered the tension mounting while there was as yet no water, mounting until at last in April the wind changed from south to north.

Then as revelation two, the water, triggered our rush—precipitating us onto the stage itself, with our tent and our watch station—the word flashed around: a sighting! And by that quiet stage, split right open to show those singing miles of glitter and ripples before us, appeared the third revelation, the WHALE. It was spring itself, not as birdsong, not as budding greenery, but surrounded by the white ice and rising from within the mystery of the warm current of the ocean: spring, bursting upon us in the shape of a vast, warm mammal. Before long the village saw it harpooned, bombed, hauled dead upon the stage, glittering black. We saw it displayed, disrobed, dismantled, down to its peculiar naked skull.

And then the RETURN. The return of the skull to the water took place, reintegrating death and darkness, ice, water, and the living soul of the mammal, all resolved at the end under the midnight twilight of those endless days. Now at the time that I was looking at the photographs, the very stage had melted into thin air, leaving not a rack behind; the very earth was changed, and we'd lost the name of action. We had months of three-wheeler land travel before us, with the glorious snowmobiles forgotten . . . until the gradual darkening and the chill days, the wind chill reminding us once again of the creative cruelty of the dark months, then the prerevelation that is the slush ice—which is the time of the whale's tail celebration. So now one sees why they celebrate, and understands what they tell. They celebrate because the ice is coming. ∎

June 7, Tuesday. The stage I thought had melted was back. Today an army of ice came in again, which was certainly not there on Monday. It was ice right up to the horizon. The south wind had simply blown floating ice in against our twelve-mile point. And I had forgotten Nalukatak, the Jumping, or Qagruq, the Arrow, or the Beaching, the prime whaling festival. This was an event that was hardly of this world but seemed to reverse everything, play on everything; and for some reason its main event took place high above ground.

Every woman in town was stitching. Annie was sewing her own purple sculptured-velvet brocade parka. She was going to look superb, quite theatrically on key. I helped her to soften and work the fur of the wolverine that Gordon had caught. Annie painted the back of the fur with red ocher collected from upriver: one must paint the back of skins red. Annie thought deeply before cutting the wolverine, so that she would not do it wrong. The most experienced Iñupiat dressmaker had this moment of thought before cutting. The animal's parka was to be converted into a human one.

Arenas of preparation for the Whaling Festival were springing up all over town. Visitors were appearing, and the men caught animals to feed them—seals and walrus. A gun went off right then, in front of the village, on a shore that was perhaps the most lively hunting ground of all. Mikigaq was being stirred, and cigarettes, oranges, and apples were being ordered, also caribou fat for Eskimo ice cream—the money was funneled in somehow. At the elders' lunch there were big encounters and greetings, hugs, cries of joy, and laughter, as long-parted relatives and friends got together.

"We played together when she was just little."

"He's my grandmother's sister's son!"

"I saw you at the elders' conference."

To experience an Iñupiat greeting and hug was a complete experience—a completing experience.

That afternoon the festival began.

17

The Whaling Festival

Qagruq, the Beaching

What was to occur during the next three days was known beforehand and took place in accordance with a well-known program, even more defined than that of the Messenger Feast. But this one was unwritten. It had never been banned by the missionaries, so it did not require—as the Messenger Feast did—a conscious revival, plus air trips, a gymnasium, and the borough mayor's official staff. This was a celebration innate to the people's way of thinking and actual way of eating. Its details were no surprise to me because I had become familiar with them from anthropologists' reports and from movies. Because of its unofficial, repeating, and foreknown program, it constituted something very stable in such a 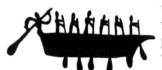 village of flux. And yet the celebration depended on whales being caught. The whale, though elusive, when it did agree to come to Ivakuk, gave the village continuity, history, and the singular cultural form of the Whaling Festival.

The Whaling Festival was an event for the qalgis. Each of the two qalgis, Qanginyiq and Ingigaqtuq, occupied its own festival ground. The two grounds were located out on the tundra on opposite sides of the village, and each qalgi hosted any visiting members of the other qalgi at all times throughout each day, concurrently, and also hosted many outside visitors. ∎

June 12, Sunday. *The First Day, the Halfway Place.* The first day was foggy. I left the house early, shivering. I first went to the Qanginyiq festival ground because Qanginyiq was my own qalgi of adoption. Only one of the five whales had been caught by a Qanginyiq member, and that was Robert Nashanik's. As I walked over the gravel in the general direction of the Qanginyiq ground, I could make out through the mist the huge jawbones that marked the ground, set up to form a open arch. At the same moment I caught sight of some figures on my right already coming up from the beach. A Honda three-wheeler was pulling along a boat perched on a sled. Several men accompanied the boat, holding it steady, and boys ran in front and behind. They stopped halfway up from the beach to the festival ground.

This "halfway" place in their parlance was important. It echoed the slow start and tentative approach in much of Inuit ritual generally. There was a halfway completed phase in Iñupiat dance, in which the first half of a stanza was played softly on the drums, and the dancers seemed merely to go through the motions, whereas the second half of the stanza was repeated loudly and danced vigorously; the same style could be noted in the gradual approach to a climax that was enacted in the principal dances of the Messenger Feast, both in the eagle dance and in the coming-out dance at the end. It was also seen in the peeking entry of the marmot in the string puppet dance at the new moon, as the marmot emerged little by little, then hid again. Among the Inuit of Canada the shaman was said to be "half-hidden" (Merkur 1985). By deduction from the positional meaning of this symbol,[1] and from Clem and Kaglik's exegesis, this was a typical Iñupiat approach to the sacred. Hesitations in face of a mystery and acknowledgments of the hard task of comprehension are repeated as a culturally emphasized part of ritual. ■

On the first day the festival had only half begun. The men were lifting the boat off the sled and upending the sled to make a stand on which to place the bow of the boat. The stern was placed on boxes to support the boat on an even keel. Facing the front, I saw how the boat was now enshrined on pedestals. This was the very boat whose skin had been painstakingly sewn by Dora and the women of the village, the very boat from which Robert's son had harpooned their whale. Quickly the men placed the paddles upright in the triumph position. Robert's son arranged his harpoon at the bow. The men drew out of a truck a flagpole displaying the stars and stripes and also the special flag of Robert's crew, carrying a picture of a whale, and they reared the flagpole upright in front of the boat. I saw what marked this particular spot on the tundra as the "halfway place." At the very bow of the boat an ancient, bare skull of a whale lay on the gravel. The men were passing the foot of the flagpole through the hole of the peculiarly-shaped skull, and the pole was then lashed to the bow of the boat. Thus the whale was honored. Clearly, this particular whale had given itself body *and* spirit to the Iñupiat.

The boat was now gallant, with paddles upright, the flags active in the wind, the boat itself raised on high, the whole plugged in to the spirit chamber of the skull below—it was the apotheosis of the boat. The enshrinement united boat and equipment and whale together with the past (the skull), the present (the boat itself), and the future (whales that would come again to good hunters and to the village that was honoring them), and it reaffirmed power to the particular qalgi on whose ground it was. Although no one actually said this at the halfway place, it had already been said in one way or the other in the processes of hunting. Now it was simply *done*.

In front of the boat the men laid boards, on which Robert's wife Dora and her women relatives placed their wooden barrels of mikigaq. This was the day for mikigaq, ripened to perfection in its five-day process, an ephemeral food that would keep no longer. Doughnuts, coffee in large thermoses, Kool-aid, and cupcakes were also ready. Crowds were gathering. When all was ready, the Nashanik family and crew lined up in front of their boat. Dora took the center and said a short prayer of gratitude for her whale. The preacher prayed and led the assembled crowd in the Lord's Prayer. Then, with the chilly mist still around us, the gathered throng sang the doxology.

As soon as the doxology was finished, a swirl of people came forward from each side and seated themselves in two crescent moons in front of the boat, visitors to the left, locals to the right, leaving an empty center. At once the women of the Nashanik family commenced to feed the people, elders first, as always. They started the rounds with the mikigaq. For this the women donned white nylon gloves, plunging them into the softened masses and bringing out drooling rags of ripe black mikigaq, at which the guests opened up plastic bags to receive them. Now the guests took tidbit mouthfuls, licking their fingers appreciatively. "Finger-lickin' good," said Ardell, grinning at me as I sat down on the gravel to receive my share. A round of doughnuts followed, then without pause, coffee and Kool-aid in styrofoam cups, all with the rushing gestures of generosity to which I was becoming accustomed. Quiet reigned except for sucking sounds and occasional bursts of laughter. After a time the people started to move off home with their goodies, and that was that for the halfway place.

I returned across the tundra, through the village, and out toward the Ingigaqtuq festival ground on the far side. There I found Clem and the other three captains at their own halfway station, with their four boats shoulder to shoulder, also enshrined. The same ritual was taking place.

In the evening the Christians organized a "singspiration" in the church. This word was obviously a combination of *sing* and *inspiration*. The singspiration consisted of sermons and hymn singing. I left early, seeing that a third of the congregation was asleep, and went home to entertain my landlady for dinner.

June 13, Monday. *The Second Day, the Day of the Flippers and the Blanket Toss.* On this day the people made an early morning trip to the graveyard to honor the dead and take them mikigaq. Afterward the people gathered to their festival ground, where the huge, arched whale jawbones formed the entryway. Inside, around the center space, were sets of rib bones at each corner of a wide square, with other bones set wider still. The boats had been brought up to the festival ground and were now beached "all the way."

This time I visited the Ingigaqtuq side first, Clem's qalgi. The path toward it and the area around the erected bones at the ground itself, in fact the whole terrain, was plain gravel, with a little grass and occasional pads of purple flowers. The men were already busy reerecting their flagpole between the two main arch bones. The single flagpole on the Ingigaqtuq side showed the flags of the four successful captains of that qalgi, topped by the flag of Clem, the flipper captain. The men also tacked up a welcome sign on the flagpole and arranged bunting from arch to arch. The four boats were drawn up in a curved line, not on pedestals this time, but tilted over on their sides, end to end, with a paddle erected between each boat. On this day the line of boats was to the south of the ground, facing the north, because the wind was from the south. The boats were set up partly as a shelter from the wind, making a place for the whaling captains to sit, and partly as the place most corresponding to the captains' roles on the sea. The theme of correspondence ran throughout the Whaling Festival—all was very close to the actual sea event of the catching of the whale, but the festival was not that event, it was its other self on land—a symbol, of course, a major one.

It was the day of the flippers. Men were beginning to seat themselves on the caribou-covered sleds that had been placed before the boat-shelters. Each crew sheltered in front of its own boat. In the middle seat of each, the place of honor, sat the captain, then, at either side of him, the harpooner, older crewmen, and one or two honored men guests. No women or children occupied boat shelters at this stage. A low camping table was set before each sled-bench, on which stood thermoses and cups. Later on Netta came and sat down beside Clem. She brought a tape recorder on which she proceeded to play Iñupiat drumming cassettes, consciously inculcating the songs of the past.

The men began putting up windbreaks of black plastic to extend the shelter further along on either side of the boats. I made my way to a plastic windbreak and sat and watched the men delivering sections of whale flipper on Honda trailers. Right in the center of the ground a number of plywood sheets were spread on the grassy gravel. Here they laid the huge flat sections of tail, two or three feet across, black on the outside with white fat inside. At the cut surfaces the white had turned an old red; these had been places of over-ripening in the ice cellar. The tail sections were those we had never seen at the dismembering of the whale because they had been cut off when the whale had first been caught, while still away on the water, and on landing they had been brought straight to the captain's wife to be stored in her ice cellar. These slabs had pre-existed as part of the huge tail itself—an extraordinary sight on the living whale as it rises, spouts, humps forward right over, then upends, joyously dancing its enormous tail in the air as a last signal. A still photograph does not capture the effect. It strikes a great sense of joy into the watcher—the tail. It seems to express emotion much as a dog's tail does, but that is a weak metaphor for such a display. The whale communicates, is telling you something.

The tail occurred as a motif throughout Iñupiat art and culture, and I was interested in the way the festival celebrated it. The clues, the pointers, were clear: they were to be seen in the Whale's Tail feasts that had occurred earlier in the year (see chaps. 5 and 12). These feasts celebrated the spine section of the tail and the stump end. The outline of a whale's tail used to be tattooed on the right wrist of a whaling captain's wife, indicating how many whales she was responsible for. In former days a visionary whale's tail was seen emerging from the mouth of the captain's wife as she walked toward the village after her shamanic act of whale-drawing. This mouth feature was added to a bone mask made by Kaglik and also appeared on the reverse side of a carved depiction of Clem's great-great-grandfather Kehuq, the man who received a shamanic gift. It was Clem himself who had carved this figure out of a walrus tusk. After first carving an effigy of the shaman-hunter Kehuq carrying a battering ball on a line, Clem turned the tusk around and carved the female aspect of Kehuq on the other side, in the form of an Iñupiaq woman, back to back with the male Kehuq. The woman figure showed a whale's tail coming out of her mouth. The association of female gender with the whale was obvious in such graphic expressions. They confirmed the saying, "The woman catches the whale."

Furthermore, in almost all bone masks the whale's tail is seen in a trompe l'oeil depicted on the face. The two eyebrows and the nose on the mask stand out in relief and are immediately seen as constituting the whale's tail (the eyebrows) and its spine (the nose). Whale and human were one in these masks.

Finally, the whale's tail was also delicious food; everyone in Ivakuk affirmed that the flipper muktuk tasted best. ■

As for the festival ground itself, right at the entrance, just before one entered through the jawbone arches that fronted the ground, there was a place for the whaling equipment. Every year the equipment was brought to the festival ground for all to see, so that this spot became a shrine for the materials of the hunt. In higgledy-piggledy piles lay grub boxes, big orange floats, sheaves of long-handled knives and choppers and hooks for the work of cutting, the harpoons themselves with the barrels attached, now empty of bomb and barb. Under those things could be seen four bloody newly-cut upper jawbones, each ten or fifteen feet long, one from each whale celebrated that year. These in turn had been heaped on top of other jawbones from previous seasons, so that the collection of bones constituted a history of Ivakuk's whaling for many years previously, with the present being uppermost literally, as well as uppermost in the mind. Annie could name the source of each jawbone, the name of the hunter, and the year the animal was caught.

Close to the equipment thus sacralized by its position were parked a large number of Honda three-wheelers belonging to the helpers. Young women kept arriving with large metal bowls containing Eskimo ice cream, that is, berries whipped up with caribou fat and flavored with seal oil. Everything on this day was frozen, not fermented or cooked. Pilot bread (hardtack) was ready to serve with the ice cream, which was the favorite savory dip.

Now Clem stood up in the middle and announced the commencement of the flipper feast (*Avariki* "whale's flippers"). Old Michael, the preacher with the trembly gait, came forward to the hunks of flipper. Then he straightened himself, firmed up, and spoke, giving thanks to God for sending the whales. He raised his arms to heaven and gave praise in Iñupiat. The people sang the doxology and immediately set to work.[2]

The middle-aged and younger men came forward and started cutting up the flipper hunks displayed on the plywood sheets, using the shorter whaling knives. They cut them as we might cut Canadian bacon, in firm slices that came out in long white ovals bordered with black. The sight of this muktuk stirred the people. Soon piles of slices were accumulating on the boards like huge, loose playing cards.

Clem stood in the middle of the boards. He picked up a thick slice of muktuk. "Netta-Atiq!" he shouted. We had come to the presentation of the muktuk, and Clem was beginning with the healers first. Netta, the oldest village healer, got to her feet and toddled forward. Here was none of the rushing forward of the giver toward the recipient, with that pushing, almost tossing motion of the earlier feasts, which occurred and recurred as a separate motif in its own right. In Avariki, the flipper rite, individual names were called, using Iñupiat names where possible. The individual then walked forward to the whaling captain, took the muktuk from his hand, bit into the muktuk, and walked back to her place with it.

Netta reached Clem, the captain and her grandson. She raised her open, withered face, received the slab of muktuk with a look of consummation, tasted it, and retired.

"Claire!" the captain called next, and Claire came forward, knowing her own prime value for the Iñupiat tribe, with a swinging step and a proud and shy head, her eyes squinched up. She received her award.

"Suellen!" he called. These three women, Netta, Claire, and Suellen, were the main healers, each a focus—in the shape of an individual—of the overarching Iñupiatness of them all. Then he called the names of the elders, then his crew, and Sam and his crew, and the other captains who helped him.

As Clem called a name he added some funny sobriquet in Iñupiat, as the laughter confirmed. Now the other captains and the wives were also calling the names. Stella, in a magnificent traditional skin coat of muskrat, decorated with family fur tags that were laden with power, glittering with domino shapes of black and white on the two long chest stripes (the walrus tusks)—the whole coat full of browns and animal colors—strode about in the center. Janet, thin and determined, called shrilly; Margie, also in her fine velvet and ruff, called kin and helpers.

I was wandering around behind the calling captains, taking video shots and trying not to get in the way of the comings and goings or the visits of young Iñupiat girls carrying ice cream to the elders, or the wandering of children.

"Edie!" I heard. It was Margie, calling my name. I had helped her clean out her house a few days before. I dashed forward, forgetting that the videocamera was on, thereby causing it to take various shots of the gravel. I went and hugged Margie, then received the fine oval of muktuk she was holding out to me. Yes, I must taste it. I did so. Belatedly remembering the camera, I trained the close-up on the muktuk so that strangers would know what it looked like.

Very moved, I went to the side. The flipper of the whale came even to me because I had been in that circle of willingness, willing to be bound to others in the bonds of the collective good—the bonds that grew the village together person by person in a concrete unity: the fleshly unity of the whale.

The gifting continued. All the helpers received their muktuk; then it was time for the rest of those present at the Ingigaqtuq qalgi side to have theirs. Bristol visitors were called up in a group to receive muktuk, and the other villages also in groups. Finally the muktuk giving was completed.

I tried to analyze this particularizing process, yet when I tried, the work of objectifying began to spoil the scene as I remembered it. What I tried to say was this: here at the point of greatest distribution, when eventually everyone without exception was going to receive some muktuk, there was a turning back from the general to the particular. That small piece of specialty whale possessed a little of the power of the whole whale. Each special person was part of the whole village, confirmed and consolidated by this rite in his or her special Iñupiat place. The individual had to take an active step to qualify for a slot in the collective pattern. There had to be a response to the call by an act of will, which then constituted a positive sign of respect. The call was from the generosity of the whale. The eating was like a communion with the spirit of the whale and at the same time an acceptance of assigned membership.

But I could not bring this symbol out of its flatness into reality, nor make it give depth to my narrative. Maybe I could, though, if I went back in time and viewed the whole year's story. Then the stepping forward might come alive. So I looked back at the year's whaling process. I could see how the gradual gathering and collectivizing of effort had accelerated and had widened village solidarity through time, from the simple biological family over the winter, from which small center a solitary hunter would depart to catch a caribou, to the first stages of widening, implicit in the plans made by the family for the whaling season—"Shall we run a boat?" Then, "Whom shall we have in the crew?" At this point the captain's wife went over in her mind all the relatives of the two of them and began to canvass for their assistance. The range of interaction was now concretely widening. The official meetings of whaling captains, the weapons workshop, and the skin sewing groups widened it further. Then the newly formed wider units, the crews, left home and took up camp positions on the ice for the hunting. Family structure stretched and changed owing to these highly liminal, betwixt-and-between circumstances. Then within this liminal time, the event of the year took place: the coming of the whale, one being that was going to feed the entire village. To strike the whale, one smart individual was needed, the harpooner. But he had to be backed by his crew and the other boats, complete with their harpooners, for one bomb rarely finished the whale. Down on the ice factions were forgotten. Any boat in the village would offer to back up a boat that had made the first successful strike. Then the tradition of eight boats to tow in the whale came into play, so we saw fifty or sixty men acting in unison, their boats in tandem, towing in the forty-ton beast. At the edge of the ice the entire village turned out to haul it in. And on that occasion all comers were fed some preliminary muktuk. For the cutting, precise meat division rules were followed, now codified by the Alaska Eskimo Whaling Commission. These rules basically gave rewards to the principal crew and the subsidiary ones in strict order. After that the custom of delivering muktuk to the elders was carried out. And in the period after the catch the village sense of unity remained, for the Whaling Festival was coming.

Everyone knew that all would receive a share at the Whaling Festival, especially if one of the captains had caught his first whale. And so we come back to the particular point on this day when the focus turned from the all to the one, to each named person. In a sense the unity was now sufficient as a safety arena in which the power of the individual could be recognized. That exact tip of the tail flipper—it was the exact thing done by the individual that merited its presentation. All was exactitude. You heard the name, the voice of the whaling captain; you answered. It was a matter of precise knowledge, consciousness, and particularity. ∎

I went home for a short rest, then returned for the next event, the blanket toss. Now the men dragged Clem's boat skin into the center of the ground. Clem was giving away his boat skin as well as the entire whale itself because the whale was his first. In fact, anything he possessed could be demanded by the villagers. He was even a little nervous about his TV set. Flipper captains had been known to allow their TV sets to be taken, but all that happened to Clem's was that it went on the blink. As for his boat skin, it was going to be used for the blanket toss, and afterward anyone could use its tough material for soles on mukluk boots.

Clem's brother and cousin were occupied in spreading the boat cover out on the ground. The sewn skin piece was long in shape and tapered at each end. They had to cut it and resew it to make it into a square. It was certainly a man's job to cut that iron-strong seal skin, now dry and still showing traces of the old hidden seams made by the women. The sewing, too, was going to be different. It was the men themselves who were going to essay the task, not with a needle (which would have a hole in it), but with an awl, with a single sharp point.

A couple of men held the two edges to be sewn so that they were overlapping each other. The pieces stood up like a wall beside them. On the shady side of the wall of skin stood another man with an awl and a length of very tough sinew, so thick that you could actually sharpen the end with a knife. This man pierced a hole in the two thicknesses of skin with his awl and poked the point of the sinew through. A fourth man this side of the "wall" was waiting for it. He grasped the emerging sinew and pulled it through. Then he in his turn pricked a hole with his awl a little higher up and afterward inserted the point of the sinew. All the men began to shake.

"Ever seen a sperm whale?" said the man as he inserted his

point. They rocked about in crazy laughter, howling delightedly. Even my videocamera shook. Gradually, interrupted by occasional giggles, they sewed the two pieces together into one stiff blanket ten feet square. Then they fitted rope handles all around the sides of the "blanket."

Now the people were gathering to the center of the festival ground. The stronger ones came forward and grasped the rope handles. The drummers in Clem's party started their tossing songs. Soon an entire square of people were gathered, beginning to tug on the handles and make the blanket rise and fall, rise and fall. There was a jostle, and Clem climbed onto the blanket and went into the middle, where he stood well balanced. They called, "One!" and pulled. "Two!" and pulled, then "Three!" Everyone gave an enormous tug, and Clem went flying into the air stiff-legged—he was not jumping; he was lifted by the propulsion of forty pairs of hands. There was laughter and a scream of joy at his ascent. He hovered, high aloft in his brilliant blue captain's jacket, levitated and galloping upon the blue sky with his legs, a big man, supremely happy. Then *whump!* He fell. Clem was still on his feet, head up, triumphant. They started pulling and sent him up again, and again. "You can pull a person up to heaven in the blanket toss," Silas told me. The sense of the collective was obvious. It was by means of all of them that one could soar.

Now Margie was supposed to go up. She had never done it before and was goggling with terror. Netta and her sisters-in-law gave her much advice and friendly encouragement. "Hold your legs stiff. Come down standing up straight."

"Cm'on Margie, you can do it," was heard all around the square. Margie struggled onto the blanket. She was carrying a large paper bag full of candy—this was because she was the mother of a little boy, little Luther. The source of all maleness, as well as of the whale, was the woman. She stood with scared eyes in the middle of the blanket, holding her bag of candy.

"One! Two! Three!" and they tossed her on high. At the zenith she contrived to tear open the bag and fling the contents everywhere.

"*Arrigaa!* Great!" Immediately this was a chance for the elders because only the elders might grab the candy. Abandoning my camera, I rushed to the place where Annie and Vera and Ruth and Helen and Agatha and Piluq were down in a scrimmage. I was a bit late in the day, as usual; the women's hands were already full of goodies, and Ruth was grabbing candy from all around me. I promptly sat down—I was confident I must have landed on some of it. Ruth began scrabbling under my behind—we were convulsed with laughter. But I sat firm. Carefully I removed three wrapped candies. [This story, like many of my foolish performances, became one that the Iñupiat loved to pass around.]

Meanwhile, Margie had survived and was up in the air again with a bag of bias bindings, zippers, cigarettes, even playing cards. After these had descended, a packet of yard goods flew through the air, then a toilet bowl brush; there were screeches of delight at this one, and Madeline, the clown, fielded it with a running catch, to the satisfaction of all. Margie had done the necessary.

Suellen came next and mounted the blanket, Suellen the healer, big and capable, wearing a magnificent parka and a royal blue crocheted cap. "One! Two! Three!" and up she went, with her healing hands neatly balancing the air. She landed triumphantly.

"All *right!*" she exclaimed with joy. And so it went on, Dick Kuper performing a veritable Iñupiat dance forty feet above our heads; then some boys who turned somersaults in the air before landing. Netta was tossed very gently—she was seventy-eight, after all—with her legs set wide like sticks, her bright blue parka flaming against the blue of the sky, and her determined gray hair awry and jolly. She too came down safely. I handed the videocamera to my ten-year-old friend so that she could take pictures from the top of a whale bone stanchion. Then I shyly pushed my way through the tossers and scrambled into the middle of the blanket.

"Hold your legs stiff!" they shouted. "Just balance. Don't try to jump." They tossed and I rose a few feet, then fell ignominiously on one side.

"Ha. Try again." They tossed and I fell on the same elbow. Ouch, that hurt. I crawled out. Okay, whatever? I had done it.

What exactly was happening at the blanket toss? Why was it the elders who could grab the candy? Was this another function of the respect due to elders, and anyway what did that imply? The elders did not have the jobs; the modern system tended to push them out on the sidelines. But I remembered that when I needed to obtain permission to attend the festival and videotape it, it was the elders to whom I was instructed to apply, not City Hall. This festival, with its qalgi system, was entirely Iñupiat. The civic authorities had no say in its running whatsoever. The presentation of whale meat to the elders, the right to the candy, all showed a turning around of the generations, having the effect of reattaching the present to the past and recreating the continuity of the culture, a culture deeply involved with the life-and-death matter of whaling, a death matter that I sensed at the weapons workshop. The present then creates the past, and I had a suspicion that the future out there somewhere was busy creating the present. (That is why Western, ultramodern, invented rituals, with no sense of the past at all, invented by us here and now, and not by some spirit agency coming into our heads from the future or the past, are so empty and lifeless.) In the blanket toss, when the young mother ascends and flings out candies, she is the embodiment of the future. She performs the act of "throwing objects upon chance"—a phallic act, but also echoing the chance element involved in all reproduction—projection, ejaculation, expulsion, "out from the body" and "into the future"—the operating principle of reproduction. The throwing, also an act of chance, is thus of the nature of the future, but the recipients are the old, the elders, grabbing vigorously to hold the future they will see when they are reborn into a new child in the community. When Joanna eventually died, the next child in the Kasugaq family was named Joanna. Here the Iñupiat custom of naming for an ancestor effects, in a peculiar way, the transference of the soul of the ancestor into the new child. The choice of a name is more a matter of a collective, nonritualized divination than it is vague supposition or guesswork. By such divination parents learn the name that will successfully bring about the transference.

About the blanket toss, there were many levels of meaning. Some Iñupiat said that people were tossed up so that they could see whales far away, but others denied it. There was also a sense that the toss, "the jumping," was an act of joy, a celebration of the hunter and what he brought. Most often the people said, "We hold the festival to honor the whale so that it will come again." I myself used Victor Turner's method for unearthing the meaning of a symbol by looking into the culture for other contexts where the same symbol is used—his "positional level of meaning." (A dominant symbol seems to have the power of refraction through many aspects of a culture. The positional method attributes certain details of power to a symbol because the wider ethnographic material appears to show such power. Here we are following a free-floating culture item wherever it leads. Furthermore, I am looking at the action and effectiveness of a ritual item, rather than regarding it as static and structural. It is more like the study of bodily processes than the study of anatomy, which is the uncovering of structures.

Thus, I saw that the dominant whale motif, to which the blanket toss and throwing of candy were related, appeared universally at whaling time in the constant gesture, a rising, bowing, and dipping forward of the curved hand, accompanied by a happy smile. This, as all knew, was the whale's rising for air, a soul-stirring sight in the eyes of every seagoing Iñupiaq. The same throwing or tossing motif with hints of the whale's spout appeared, as described previously, in many aspects of the festival life; here it was seen in the fizzy, bubbly mikigaq (the fermented meat) and the whipped-up Eskimo ice cream. It was in the sexual joking about the "sperm whale" while the men were sewing the blanket. Was the erection of paddles and flags and whale bones on the festival ground also connected with this? Spouting, fizzing, objects rising into the air, erection, orgasm, childbirth, all were motifs present in the culture, but they were not verbally connected to the blanket toss. ■

June 14, Tuesday. *The Day of the Cooking.* When I arrived at the Ingigaqtuq ground, I found the men changing the boats from the south side to the north because the wind had changed and was coming from the north. I helped carry the windbreak supports from the south to the north. Will Pingasut offered me some coffee from his station in front of his boat and pointed out the owners and positions of the boats. Although two of the captains were Jacksons and cousins, they did not place their boats next to each other; in fact, theirs were the furthest apart. As the people gathered, the visitors tended to cluster at the village end of the ground. Now another long windbreak was erected on the south side, where the women started to do their cooking. The division of labor here resulted in the separation of the women's and men's sectors on the festival ground. Behind the women's windbreak was a busy scene. Honda three-wheelers were arriving in dozens, loaded with the most important equipment, particularly the stoves that had once stood inside the tents down on the ice, now set up on the land with their chimneys anchored by wire. The women crews each had a station on the lee side of the windbreak, facing the sea, in positions corresponding to the position of the boats and the men. Each cooking crew placed its stove opposite its station and a little way off because of the smoke. Between the stoves and the women's stations lay plywood board floorings, one for each crew. These became huge cutting boards, on which the men began to deposit heavy loads of meat for the cooking pots.

Margie, at the far end, was getting her corner in order. She had acquired two large Coleman stoves and had dough already rising in a two-foot-wide metal bowl. I turned to her big wood stove with its chimney and helped fuel it, using driftwood and seal fat as in the days on the ice. Margie was going to cook on this stove using two thirty-two-quart cooking pots at a time. Clem came up on his Honda, pulling a trailer laden with whale heart and kidney, black whale meat, walrus meat, seals, ducks, and also lagoon ice for water. I began to help Madeline cut up meat on Margie's board: Madeline was helping Margie because of a distant relationship. We got to work. Some of that muscle meat came in huge, anomalous lumps, so I had to take my ulu knife and work around the worst cartilage patches and slimy sliding joint areas and cut four-inch lumps that would go into the pans. Not skillful at letting the knife continually slide away from me in a drawing motion and thus make the knife do the work for me, I soon developed a blister on my palm. But I didn't mention it.

"You're my *boyur*," said Madeline, laughing. She meant the boy who does the fetch-and-carry jobs down on the ice. I grinned. I'd be the boyur, any time. After a while the anthropologist took over from the boyur, and I went wandering up the line of crew women to see what was happening. The Pingasuts had hauled up a large section of beluga whale. I greeted Stella, who was busy cooking portions of her delicious round whale—a small one, and tasty. At the far end I drank a cup of tea, then left the cooking line and went to visit the men in the tilted-over boats. Afterward I wandered back to the cooks behind the windbreak. I had forgotten my meat-cutting job. I found my way to Madeline's board. All the meat was finished and gone.

"Boyur, you've got the sack," she said and raised a laugh from the cooks around her. "Where was you?" I grinned and showed her my blister.

"Ah-zaa!" she said surprised.

This whole festival was turning me upside down, somewhat. Margie was busy with her Coleman stoves, which now were loaded with huge skillets of sizzling oil, in which bounced golden doughnuts. You could smell the sugar and the dough freshly plumped up and browned—an irresistible aroma in the open air.

"Have one," said Margie. I did. [I could do with one as I write.] I helped her shape new doughnuts out of the dough, slip them into the sizzling oil, and fish them out when done. We must have cooked hundreds by the time we were finished, and all the time the young girls were taking hundreds of cooked meat portions and doughnuts and coffee to the crowd. We stuffed ourselves that afternoon until we could eat no more.

Meanwhile, the blanket toss continued, and races were organized on the tundra beyond the festival ground. Afterward Ingigaqtuqs and Qanginyiqs were lined up against each other in a tug of war, using a length of whaling rope. I took my place on the Qanginyiq side, and in this event we won.

When I went over to the Qanginyiq festival ground, it was the same. Dora, vast and splendidly dressed, was running the show. I saw her screeching delightedly from forty feet up in the blanket toss.

After Robert and Dora had performed, the fat Madeline got into the blanket. "Hey, we have to toss a whale," they complained, and gave it to her in good measure. Was this some exciting symbol of the real meaning of the blanket toss? Was this really the great leap of the whale, appearing from nowhere, spouting wide on the ocean? Neither I nor the Iñupiat were in a serious enough mood to answer that. Maybe it would come up later.

After a while the stiff skin blanket was laid down on the ground in front of the boat to make a carpet for dancing. The drummers sat within the boat, busily tapping the under-rims of their drums, "clack-clack," causing the humming of the drumskins. Robert performed his dance with his habitual air of modesty and firmness— and also amusement. He was the classic modest whale catcher. Old Seth, with the eyebrows, stomped and jerked, and then Madeline came on, wearing a huge pair of silver-gray oven gloves like bird's wings and did her mock eagle dance. Heads were shaken hopelessly. "That Madeline!"

How did it all end? I was by now dizzy with something like sunstroke and simply went home to bed. The end was an all-village dance in the school gym, an event that I was told went off like a dream. I saw the same final event myself three years later and witnessed the factions sitting amicably together. Ed Tukumavik moved up and allowed Clem a central place. Sam Kasugaq was sitting on Clem's other side, and he and Clem were joking together.

In the gym food was being presented, not on a qalgi basis, but to everybody. And after it was over at 1:30 A.M., they opened the doors of the hot, lighted gym, and we went out—into plentiful sunshine and coolness, into a world of long shadows and a bright blue sky.

The Pattern of the Whaling Festival. One could point to a neat web of symbols making a statement about men as hunters, practical and central to society, versus women's place in the festival, the festival being a representation of the sea hunt performed on land.

After the **spring** whaling on the **sea** is over, and **summer** has come, the boats are pulled up onto the festival ground, the **land**. The paddles, once used in the sea down below, are set up erect. **Men** occupy the **center** of the ground with their boats, the boats that it had once been essential to keep **level** on the sea; now they are **upturned**. **Women** occupy the **periphery**. **Raw** whale parts are served by the **men, calling individuals to them. Cooked and fermented** whale parts are served by **women, approaching the recipients collectively.** The boat **skin**, sewn by women when **wet**, is taken off the boat **frame** that was originally made by men. The skin, now **dry**, is sewn by men to make the blanket. The skin of the blanket was formerly designed as a hull to keep the hunters **safe**, down on the surface of the **sea**, now it is used to provide a spice of **danger**, tossing people up in the **air**.

All these distinctions appear:

> spring/summer
> sea/land
> below/above
> men/women
> center/periphery
> level/upturned
> raw/cooked and fermented
> individuals/collectivity
> frame/skin
> dry/wet
> safety/danger
> sea/air
> down/up

This kind of patterning appears to follow the anthropological theory of structuralism, based on the universality of binary oppositions and the way they symbolize society. The chief of these oppositions in structuralist theory is *nature* versus *culture,* a conclusion drawn by Lévi-Strauss (1963) about peoples living in dangerous tropical forests, possessing a mythology that seemed to sanctify their advance from wild nature to culture. But was the Whaling

Festival culture and the hunt nature? The pairs did not line up. I tried to discuss these oppositions with my Iñupiat friends, Clem, Jim, Naluq, and Annie. But there were no takers. The list of oppositions, especially women and men and sea and land, did not seem to matter to them. But when I gave up and repeated what they had told me about the purpose of the festival being the honoring of the whale, they warmed to me.

So essentially, a structuralist theory did not suit the Iñupiat. Nor did an interpretation of the festival as a covertly political act of opposition to the Whites, though Clem knew he needed to guard against the encroachment of the Whites so that the whale would continue to be honored. Such a political interpretation was the kind set out by Taussig in his book *Shamanism, Colonialism, and the Wild Man* (1987).

As for honoring the whale, what is entailed in that? Are we able to map out a theory that the Iñupiat themselves might recognize?[3] And further, should we stop at "Iñupiat theory?" Is there some theory of our own that might be inspired enough to bridge the gap—like the shaman crossing his precarious bridge—between Iñupiat culture and our understanding?

First, for matters that the Iñupiat would recognize at once, such as the values that are sought before and during the festival—Which issues are these? Which most engage the participants? First and foremost is *giving*, the ability to feed the village until it is absolutely satiated; then sewing a fine parka, and the particular quality of the mikigaq and doughnuts; for the men, the unboasted fact of having brought in whales, with credit due not to them but to the intent of the whale in recognition of the goodness of their wives; then their daring at the blanket toss; and afterward the exactness and address of their dancing. The quality of each particular whale as food and the skill in the processing frequently came to the fore in gossip. And behind all that was the story of the catching of each animal—each story went around the village and was savored.

The festival purpose that meant most to the people was honoring the whale, in order to bring it back the following year. The Iñupiat did think about it. As the Ivakuk people said, if you catch an animal and treat its parka (body) with respect, it will come again. The festival clearly used the parka, the meat, in an honorable way; it celebrated it above all things. The people prayed at the start of each phase of the festival—even using Christian prayer because the whale meant so much. Prayer put the stamp of spirit meaning on the whale in an unmistakable way, and at the same time the peculiar spirit meaning of the whale rendered the Christian prayer itself ineluctably Iñupiat. Eating, the other major act, completed the cosmological cycle and fulfilled the purpose of the whale's coming.

The whale brought into being an entire moral universe. It could hear what we said in the house. It liked a white boat and a clean ice cellar. It wanted to come to a good wife. The initiative was with the whale. This is the opposite of the ethos of many Western sports hunters, who view hunting as a contest, whose ambition is to defeat the animal and bring it low—"man triumphant," as illustrated in old photographs of a White man in India wearing a solar topee, with his foot on the neck of the tiger he has killed. Walens (1981, 163, 1987) and Sharp (1994) show that American Indians sense that they gain a spirit from the animals who have given themselves to the hunter, and that to give the spirit was the animals' purpose. The same ethos ran through the Ivakuk Whaling Festival.

But the Whaling Festival took off in a curious way, not directly connected with the moral. Those odd patterns noted above were actually there, to be seen on the ground, and they were interesting, however much the Inupiat took them for granted. The phenomenon in one sense looks like the structure of the community set at play, not law. It appears to be "the game of form." The structures of society regarded as social law, as Victor Turner (1969) said, can become oppressive, top-heavy, until communitas breaks in and renews genuine social ties. One may follow these processes among high civilizations. But as art the forms can become joyous, freely elaborating, exuberant, the apparent opposite of themselves. This kind of elaboration is germane to the genre of play—it originates in play. The whaling and its festival at Ivakuk exemplify this process. All of it has to do with superabundance, with the Gargantuan whale, in the Rabelaisian mood. One might indeed capture this structure, so called, for communitas and get it drunk or mad, as Shakespeare's favorite characters did to Bottom or Malvolio. The same superabundance combined with elaboration is seen depicted in the baroque style in Western art, in Mexican churrigueresque, in the shaman's curlicues carved in the ancient spiral motifs found by archeologists at Ivakuk, in the complex crowns of the old shaman kings of Korea, in Navajo sand paintings, in Huichol wool paintings, in Aztec codices, in the *veve* arabesque floor designs of Voudon and the *riscado* floor sketches of Brazilian Umbanda, in

African circumcision masks, and in the many different, particular-ized, and extraordinary extravagances of oriental art. The style, if not the iconography itself, which may have its own rich meaning, is complex exuberant jollification, productive of dizziness. The mood may sometimes be triggered by drugs or the art may be simply the depiction of a shamanic vision.

Thus, I might regard the Whaling Festival as an event that does indeed throw up patterns, reflections, and opposites, as many festivals do. I begin, like the Iñupiat, with the original spirit of the whale. The spirit meaning that flows from the whale spins off elaborations of so-called structural significance, scintillating, re-fracting, rearranging, or inverting sometimes, evolving a style cor-responding to verbal and grammatical and logical forms that is all its own, creating neat, kaleidoscopic effects not only of binary but of sextuple, multiple discriminations. These are focused and fall into place, although only the rough outlines are found in everyday society and nature. In the Whaling Festival the village sees its men on one side and its women on the other, whereas these are so of-ten mingled in everyday life. It sees the elders gathered and feeds them first, the young serving them: old and young. The difference between sea and dry land is of the very essence in this festival. It consists of the actual flowery ground beneath our feet, not "good to think" in the mind, to quote the structuralist Lévi-Strauss (1963), but experienced in the body. Why would we need to talk about that? We showed our joy by simply rushing to the festival, we were *doing* the whale and its coming. And high/low, the up-right paddles and the blanket toss, are echoes of a peculiarly Alaskan Eskimo idiom, that of throwing. These are ephemeral phenomena coming into existence and fading away again, part of the special character of celebration. As for any nature/culture dis-tinction, it appears that the Iñupiat celebrate exactly the opposite of any such distinction: they celebrate something like Lévy-Bruhl's (1985) law of mystical participation. Nature and culture are one, the reverse of being distinct from one another; they participate one with the other. The shamanic view, like Buddhism, includes all sentient beings together, even mountains and lakes, so that ideas of separation, fear, and protection from nature-as-an-enemy do not come into the picture. Connectedness does. What I am saying is a fundamental matter and takes us out of the realm of psychology and logical laws to the realm of the spirit and play. It takes us, furthermore, out of the realm of metaphor because the festival is not held in order to represent the whale, but actually to honor it. And this is different.

Victor Turner (1974, 202) approached the essence of celebrations by way of liminality theory. Celebrations are liminal rituals, in the betwixt and between of normal life—in which anything can happen, in which you indulge in the oddity of extremes and contrasts and pairings and reflexive discriminations that are fun for fun's sake. These are *loved*, not *feared*, not ordered from above but indulged in below, wallowed in, relished: explored and elaborated, not immutably given and dreaded. Each year the mikigaq could be different. The ferment is alive; the festival bubbles up yearly in its own way. It *transpires*, to use Ronald Grimes's phrase about true ritual (personal communication). One cannot avoid the mikigaq—slobbery, carnal, delicious—getting it out of the barrel is like a hand exploring sex; it is black and odorous, flavored with a bouquet that is something between champagne and fish, and a lot better than oysters on the shell.

The heightened intensity of the festival becomes obvious. The boats are raised painstakingly at the Halfway Place, literally enshrined, with their paddles erect, revered in the liminal halfway place. The flags are gallant in the stiff breeze, each designating a whale. The boats are not yet fully advanced to the festival ground, but they are hailed with the women's mikigaq food, given by women whose hands rummage in deep, bloody barrels. Then on the day of the Flippers, the boats are taken to the place of the jawbones, foursquare, in pairs, framing the sky, and the captains give us clean-cut frozen muktuk, the best there is. All the tundra is now patterned with sky-marking upright motifs: with flags upright, paddles upright, whale bones upright. The boats are on their sides in a hedge barrier (not the barrier of a pressure ridge of ice this time).

On the Day of the Cooking, the stove chimneys are upright and wired into position, there for outdoor cooking, not indoor, not in the village, not on the ice nor on the ocean. The women cook heart, stomach, intestines, and kidneys, blobby objects in a big mass, soft "women's" organs, feeding everybody. This time the men make a blanket out of the boat skin, and it is done when the skin is dry, not wet as it was when originally fitted on the boat: it is punctured with awls and fastened together with thongs, not sewn wet with skillful halfway sewing in two rows to insure waterproofness. Now, firmness for the blanket is essential, male firmness, for the men and captains, the drummers, and the leapers tossed by the tossers, the inner core of the village. This is fun, and it is done not on the Arctic Ocean but on the tundra, on land. There, the waves tossed; now there are human-made waves. The leapers are happy, super-skilled, with that little bit of danger that can be created in a time of play, not under the rule of necessity.

We see an increase of domesticity at the festival, but none of it is ordinary domesticity. The cooking scene is a replica of ice-camp life, the nomadic hunter's world, using the same stove and pipe, except that the pipe is anchored with wire, just as the tent was anchored with rope to enormous chunks of ice; they use the same pots and pans, the same Coleman stoves, and doughnuts are made in the same way. All this, the very same women's work of cooking as back-up for the hunters, is now carnivalized.

The Whaling Feast is the elaborate distillation of connectedness. Sea matters have been brought *to* the land, the whale is literally incorporated *into* the people. All those particular features of the society, the personalities newly highlighted by the calling of names, the kaleidoscopic ornamentation of parkas, the odd regularities of custom, are brought together and finally united in the last all-village dance, where all partake of the whale.

Is this a legitimate way to describe it? The fact that the people themselves do not think in the literary terms that I am using is a trouble. Is there a legitimate style, a people's style, as in the publications of the borough that consist of literal transcriptions of Iñupiat stories, a kind of folklore? Is the private world of the anthropologists an illegitimate enterprise, with its structuralism, processualism, postmodernism, critical anthropology, political correctness, constructionism, deconstructionism, interculturalism, radical empiricism, feminism—terms that seem so foreign to the big crowd, the events, and the laughter? I have only looked at what I could see and become carried away by it. The people themselves are totally enthusiastic about the festival—that we have in common. Still, we anthropologists have eaten the apple of Eden and like it, and will go on eating it.

Where their views and mine do converge is in the matter of the spirit. Here there is space to turn around; it is here that the whole Iñupiat story is tied together, the practical to the visionary. I do not term this *analysis,* or just *meaning,* but the reporting of facts at a different level. At the Whaling Festival the whale comes; it comes to the whole village through the agency of the women and the men. It comes to the land. That is why the people are tossed on the boat skin, leaping higher than anything else on land, because the whale has come. *It,* the whale, is leaping. It organizes and reorganizes everything; it particularizes, distinguishes, focuses, gives coherence, as when the laser beam makes the hologram. It breaks out in dancing. As the Iñupiat say, if they respond and dance, the animals come to them. Then the circle of the cosmos moves; it circulates. Adding this spirit element is like adding the square root of minus one to certain mathematical problems: everything falls into place and the equation works out. ∎

18

The Shaman's Four-Day Syndrome

June 18, Saturday. Clem was talking to an Iñupiaq woman scholar who was visiting during the period of the festival. The conversation began to focus on the publication of material on Iñupiat culture. The Iñupiat scholar wanted me to understand how the Iñupiat felt about the words "story," "legend," and "fable." She resented the use of the words in connection with the Iñupiat past.

"Clem and I are prehistoric man," she said, "We're directly descended from prehistoric man. There's also protohistory. There's prehistory and protohistory, see? Oral history is actually protohistory. It's valid even though it isn't written down. Don't call it story. That makes it looks as if it isn't true. And when you write what Iñupiat say"—she emphasized this to me— "put it into good English, don't write down our mistakes. We speak pure Eskimo. It should be translated into pure English. What often happens is that we're made to look ignorant."

"Okay, I promise you I won't use those disparaging words, and I'll write the conversations in pure English."

[Unfortunately my English, pure or otherwise, could never do justice to the lilt of speech of the Iñupiat, their plaint-like tones and thoughtful words, lively and to the point. It came out a little, though, in the transcriptions of the taped account of Netta's *word* and in the transcribed extracts from Claire's life history, below.]

June 21, Tuesday. At 3:00 A.M., exactly at midnight at that longitude,[1] I took a photograph of Annie's house in radiant, slanting sunlight, so as to make records at both solstices, the other being at noon on December 21 in the golden line of twilight.

June 23, Thursday. *Claire's Experiences.* Claire came in to visit, and over a cup of herb tea with honey in it, she began to talk about her childhood. After describing her babyhood she said, "When you come to think of it, I could go all the way back to about a month and a half. All those years I could flash back"—she snapped her fingers, her warm-olive face amazed, telling me. "I could go way back and remember every word they said to me. If I just think about it, it comes back to me; picture that house—I could just feel it, I'd be there—as I described visiting and listening to an old lady. I used to rub her back. I didn't realize she had back trouble and that the only time she felt good was when I was there and had been massaging her. 'Yeah,' she'd say. 'Go like that.' And then I'd get my hands and press. I remembered her house and can describe it. Not long ago an old lady told me, 'That was my mother.' She said, 'What I want to know is what you did when you used to rub her back for her. Describe the house. No, you can't!'

"But I did. I was only two years old. My mother, grandmother, and great-grandmother were all healers, and I learned from them. I remember healing someone when I was four, just like my daughter healed my stomach when she was four.

"I can't really say I learned it. I feel it. I get the symptoms from those people. I—they get sick. That's the most important part, the feelings, and I know it, I always felt it. I could sense it. I have to pray about it a lot of times, though. I don't do the healing myself, I know the good Lord gave it to me, so I'm not going to take all the credit for it." And then she said with great seriousness, "I just never doubt it, too. I *don't doubt* and I *refuse* to doubt. It's one of the main things.

"Like the other day: I was getting bad symptoms in my side, in my stomach. I lay down but I couldn't get it away. And the next day a woman came and asked me to work on her. She had all the symptoms that I had the night before I saw her. I couldn't eat and didn't want to eat; I wasn't really nauseated, but I was uncomfortable. And here she was thinking about me all the time. I get all her symptoms every time I work on her. It's more powerful when they think about me. I was affected really easily by that, badly affected. Sometimes I just feel for them to come, and I know they will. You talk about somebody and they'll walk right in. It's happened like that so many times; I always know it. But I could block it off."

All this time I was making assenting noises and pouring out more tea and honey. Claire's voice and her speaking style were inseparable from the subject matter, and her experiences came in a series of vivid pictures. The style itself spoke of great self-confidence, such as one encounters in the personal histories of exceptional people. "*I* dared to visit the old woman"—no one else. She understood speech practically from birth. The subject matter and style were all one with the flow of knowledge, "I just knew." It was a life that unfolded by its own dynamic. The unitary principle, her consciousness of herself, was very strong.

At different stages of Claire's life she had experienced certain episodes—possibly four of them—that psychologists in our culture might term *fugue* or even *psychosis*—but these episodes did not derive from psychosis. They appeared to be the classic irruptions of shamanic experience, just as the ancient Iñupiat knew them, typically lasting four days. In early times they were characterized by meeting with something fearful, a spirit of the dead or of an animal, one that first afflicted the incipient shaman, then changed and became a helper.

The account of Claire's first recorded episode was given by a friend of hers, a White woman whom I met in Fairbanks. In about 1970 Claire was in Anchorage in an expensive hotel, alone for four days, for reasons unknown.

"There she had some kind of transformation," said Claire's friend, looking disturbed. "She told me on the phone—I was at the airport—she told me she'd had some kind of revelation about me. There were certain things that would happen. A person who didn't know Claire's powers would think she'd gone crazy. It was glossolalia. That was a bad time for Claire."

The friend bent over her coffee thinking. "I don't know what Claire went through in that hotel all by herself for four days."

In 1984, when Claire was not doing much healing, she had another episode, a very bad one. Claire would continually see a devil figure in her peripheral vision. At one time in the bad phase Claire uttered a whole lot of blah-blah-blah nonsense words. It was glossolalia again. It greatly upset her relatives. Claire told them irritably, "Don't be like that, you don't think I am anything, do you? I can't help it, it comes to me." But at the end of the four-day episode Claire was able to pray to Jesus again, and afterward her healing power was stronger. She appealed to Jesus to be her helper spirit—the obverse of Satan. This was the same switch from dangerous spirit to helpful spirit that shamans experienced in the pre-Christian days.

In the fall term of 1987 Claire and Rebecca, the American Indian school secretary, were studying anthropology together by teleconference.[2] In response to an essay question, Rebecca pseudonymously used Claire's case to illustrate the experiences of shamans. Rebecca told me that because of her studies she was coming to realize that the personality of a shaman and healer was not like that of ordinary people and that such episodes as Claire's were not necessarily bad.

A further episode occurred during my fieldwork. On Thursday, January 14, 1988, as described in chapter 9, just before Jimmy got lost in the tundra, I found Claire lying on her couch, very depressed, in what psychiatrists term a state of fugue. She shut her eyes and would not speak. I was frightened, thinking she was angry. Four days later she was herself again. What I saw had all the hallmarks of a shamanic episode.

During a visit in 1991 yet another episode seems to have occurred. I had just arrived for the whaling festival and heard that Claire had returned from the hospital, where she had been a patient from May 28 to June 2. I went to her house.

"Where's Claire?"

"Washing dishes," said young Ann.

I approached the kitchen. A small, dark figure was at the sink, and she did not turn around.

"Claire, Claire. Look at this. I've brought you something." She still did not turn. Her gray hair was scrawny, her figure thin. I immediately thought, "An episode again? Isn't this fieldwork pitiful! My dear friend caught up in . . . something so mysterious. Okay, I have to try to understand it."

Claire peeped into the shopping bag I brought and saw peacock blue velvet for a new parka and a peacock blue zipper. She turned convulsively and flung herself into my arms. We were crying. I stroked her wild gray hair and haggard face.

"Dear Claire. You've given me everything, my sweet friend." When we recovered she told me the doctor at the hospital had given her the wrong medicine. She was really mad at him. "I'll get an attorney," she said. Now she was off all medicines and was feeling better by the minute. I wondered what the doctor thought he had prescribed the medicine for.

Claire had read what I had written about shamans and healers. "I *liked* it," she said. "I liked the comparisons [between shamans and healers]." I was delighted. Accordingly, I incorporated much of what she had read into this book.

The four-day period puzzled me. But there were other examples. Clem's great-great-grandfather Kehuq had experienced it in the course of his shaman initiation. When Kehuq was a young man, he was out on the tundra one day when he heard the sound of paddles up in the air. He looked up and saw a boat floating in the sky. It landed, and Kehuq saw in it a shaman with one big eye, who danced and gave him pleasure. The boat disappeared, and by the time Kehuq reached home he had forgotten all about it. Late that night Kehuq started up naked and left the tent for no reason. They brought him back, and for four days he was crazy and could not eat. But when he recovered, Kehuq could dance. When he did so his own spirit left him, and he was possessed by the strange shaman's spirit. Kehuq taught the people the shaman's songs and also taught them how to carve the shaman's face in wood. He was now gifted with shamanic powers himself.

Many shamans began this way, suffering a crazy period typically followed by a very successful hunting period and by healing gifts and other benefits. The shamanic experience may well be the key to the four-day syndrome.

One of Clem's brothers also had four-day episodes when he would not talk to anyone. Clem himself was familiar with the condition. Furthermore, Jean Briggs (1970, 254–55) mentions that during her fieldwork among the Inuit of Canada, the father of the family with whom she lived appeared to become withdrawn at periods, with the same moodiness and dislike of disturbance as Claire. The so-called arctic hysteria (Foulks 1972) may not be a matter of light deprivation so much as the four-day phenomenon. My own late husband, Vic, suffered black periods from time to time. We both used to note that they lasted for four days.[3] ∎

June 23, Thursday, continued. Claire now described her near-death experiences. I did not know if Iñupiat near-death experiences were of the same nature as the shaman's four-day episodes. Possibly in one sense they were.

"I died three times," said Claire. "The second time I was at first on a broad road, then I went to a narrow road. There was thunder, and a voice said in Eskimo, 'Go back! Your work is not finished on earth.'

"It was hard for me to go back because when I returned I was in pain.

"The third time there was an angel and a bright light. He said, 'If you step forward you will not go back. If you go back now, it will be the next time.' (She meant, "When this happens again, you will step forward and go into the light forever.") There was this bright light, and the angel touched my hands on both sides with the light. The healing is now stronger; I owe it only to God.

"You can see if a person's going to die. The person looks like a still boat on a still sea going forward far away. You have to bring it back and back, so that the person doesn't die."

Here the near-death experience shows the experience of the soul after the body has momentarily died. Many shamans in the old days were known to have come back from death after the same classic four days, having experienced a journey to the abode of the spirits. Perhaps Claire's "person" like a boat going far away is a clue. She does not call this "person" soul. Nevertheless, the Iñupiat word for "person" is *iñuk,* to which the word *iñua* "soul" is closely related. Clearly, we see two entities, the sick person's body—for instance, Netta Jackson's in her sickness—and that "person," leaving and going far away.

So the four-day episodes come at the will of the spirit beings and cut the ordinary person off from ordinary life. They cause the person to reassemble differently inside—like a chrysalis. The process has to do not only with the brain, but also the body. Shamans' powers as reported in the four-day examples are the work of this reassembled person.[4] To Claire and the others, the perception of these workings was a familiar thing. They *knew,* as they were never tired of telling me. Okay, I *knew* too, and I found that what I have described was not a hypothesis but a working system.

The development of a sense of such processes is the subject of this book. Spotting what was going on in the apparently random material of everyday led me to discriminate which were spirit events. So my days were like a divining basket, with objects randomly laid about. One tossed them, and they said something that communicated.

Claire reiterated that her healing was "different." Yet I do not call her healing "outside the world," "transcendent." No. That "different" world is amenable to our understanding; it is susceptible to the inquiries of the scholar of natural history; both worlds are within the purview of the researcher—but such a researcher has to have eyes suitable for what she or he is researching, and use those eyes. ■

June 24, Friday. I went down to the eastern shore with Annie to help her skin some big bearded seals, ugruk. Yesterday the ice had ridden completely away over the horizon, and today all of it was back in force. It was crowded up in bergs and hedges along the shore and also lay in shifting continents right up to the horizon. Nearby, on a small iceberg in front of a pool, sat Kaglik, with his gun at the ready. Kaglik was doing the seal catching, and Annie and I were busy preparing sealskins for next year's boat covering.

Annie and I stayed until midnight and into the early hours of the morning, seeing no darkness at all. I felt the days of total light fulfilled all my longing, completed my life. There was no night, no deprivation, no shutting out, only unbounded generosity of light all the twenty-four hours.

White ice, blue ice, gray ice with black sand on it floated on the sea, jumbled from some earlier violent collision with the shore. It could all be up and away in an hour or so. Now a man was walking a mile out on this ice, testing it with a long pole as he felt his way along. He reached a ridge, where he stood watching. I could hear sporadic shots.

[After this entry a period of absence intervened, when I was visiting St. Lawrence Island and eastern Siberia.]

August 23, Tuesday. I was due to leave Ivakuk finally in a few days. I had heard that Ezra Lowe had been in the hospital and was back. He was weakening. Sadly, a farewell visit must be made. I went to his house to say goodbye. He was sitting in a square, comfortable living room. The place had a good feeling about it.

"I built it myself," he said. "With my hands"—he flickered them modestly.

I never mentioned his illness. I said, "Will you go upriver to your camp?" I had heard this was a possibility.

"I would dearly like to. Only I have this cold." He did seem to have a lot of mucus from a cold, and a dry mouth from his medications. "It's dehydration," he explained. He was making an effort to hold himself together.

"Get them to adjust your medications," I said. "There are all kinds, and they could quite possibly alter them." He had had the cold since Sunday. [In spite of that, I heard his wife did manage to take him upriver, just once.]

He was going to have to go to Bristol for a checkup the following day, so I left him so that he could rest. I shook his hand as warmly as I could. There was a considerate, conscious personality occupying that fauve face and body.

Crossing-lines were approaching to alter both our courses. They bore down to turn him from that body, perhaps so that he could take up habitation in one of the babies of Dick Kuper and Ava, the daughter of Suellen, for these would be his great-grandchildren.[5] I departed, geographically. Two weeks later, on September 8, Ezra went on his possibly multiple ways.

Reconnecting After Absence

After the single year with the Iñupiat I returned to Ivakuk for short periods annually. When I arrived for a short visit in March 1989, I thought I knew most of the hazards. But on March 11 I awoke and the roar was all around me. I could hear a continuous rustle as if paper were tattering outside the window. I looked out. All I could see was snow rushing past horizontally from left to right in billows, in gusts, in gouts, in clouds, in waves, in uncontrolled and monstrous wafts of white, each hysterically different, each frustrated at finding a house standing in the way. The dune a foot from the window had grown, and I could see by looking down that the hollow by the wall itself was knifed deep. Just sometimes I could see the blurry outline of the next-door house twenty feet away. Nothing else. How was I going to be able to go out?

The citizens band radio at the end of the living room was full of school office messages. "Can't. Blocked in." Some teachers had apparently managed to make it to school, and a handful of high school students. The bus was not running, so the students must have walked or gone by snowmobile. I opened the door to the storm porch and then opened the further door. Yes, indeed. Nothing but a snowmobile could have driven up and over the twelve-foot drift I saw hanging across the road. The drift seemed to peak and then drop off like a cliff on the other side. I shut the door pretty quick.

Perhaps half a dozen snowmobiles passed during the course of the whole morning. The drivers must have been determined and found some way through at the side of the dunes, or made the drop like a trick cyclist. You need a trick cyclist if you go out in weather like this (the weather forces you to make jokes).

I did venture out in my parka, its ruff over my head and tied right over my nose. I tried to follow the track marks and continually had to struggle to the top of a dune, hating the drop on the other side because I didn't know where to tread. There was nowhere to tread. I sat down instead and slid heavily to the ground. Ouch. Poor old grandma. When I arrived at the store it was silent and almost deserted. All wise Iñupiat were at home with their thermostats set to 80 degrees, watching the TV. Not even the snowplow was out yet. Its driver would not be able to see to drive; he would be sure to collide with something. It was peaceful out there, and wild.

The reason I went out was this: Seth Lowe had promised to show me a curious spinning top that was used in the course of the winter solstice dance, for purposes of divination. This last winter, as a result of growing pride in their culture, they had revived the winter solstice dance.

At Seth's house the old man was rummaging in a box. He brought out a wooden thing. He had carved it himself out of pine wood. It was in two parts. Seth lifted off the upper half. This was a large, rounded, dome-shaped object, about five inches high and three inches across, with a nicely curved groove marking a vertical division as on a plum, though this had nothing to do with the working of the thing. Beneath the dome projected a three-inch peg. The other component was a sturdy, hollow handle. The peg of the dome section fitted with much space to spare into the hollow of the handle, so that the dome could spin around.

Later I saw that this was the way a traditional harpoon was constructed. The harpoon would have an eight-foot wooden shaft with a further shaft projecting from it, permanently fastened. This upper shaft was the immensely tough penis bone of a walrus. Atop that again was set a toggle made of ivory that held the hard, finely ground and sharpened slate blade. The toggle had a carved hole to accommodate the penis bone, which just fitted nicely, so that, when the harpoon was cast, the toggle blade entered the whale, the penis bone and shaft could be pulled loose from the toggle, and the whole harpoon could be safely retrieved on a line. The toggle, on a line of its own, was jerked by the hunter into a transverse position under the whale's skin, forming an anchorage that could not be tugged free. This little matter of the nonpermanent but snug fit of the toggle over the penis bone was the key to Iñupiat survival along these coasts because it had first enabled them to pull in whales. Now (as described in chapter 13) the same principle holds in the modern "darting gun" harpoon, also a thrown harpoon. Here the bomb fits loosely into the steel barrel of the harpoon and is projected or "darted" into the whale by means of a gunpowder shell. Even a bow and arrow works on the same principle, the arrow sitting loosely on the bowstring. Looking at the sketch I made from memory of the spinning top, I saw how like a pair of plummy testicles it was, with a penis below. The principles of fitting into holes and easy detachment seemed very important here. ▪

As for the spinning top, Seth pointed out that its hollow handle was pierced with a tiny hole. To spin the top a fine sinew was wound many times around the peg under the top component and threaded through the tiny hole in the handle from the inside of the handle to the outside. Then the top component, the dome with its peg and string, was fitted loosely into the hollow handle. The string was now protruding from the tiny hole. When Seth gave a sharp pull on the string, he could make the domed top spin rapidly around. The domed top was cut all over with notches, which were carved there for the insertion of duck's down feathers. At the solstice ritual this curious object was taken out, set all over with down, and spun, whereupon the domed top detached and its feathers were supposed to fly up high and all over the place. If they rose high in a big cloud, the village would catch many whales in the coming season. If not, they would not catch any. The spinning top was a kind of "will-it-happen-or-won't-it-happen" divination device. Chance was part and parcel of the spirit world, so in this sense the performance of the spinning top was the performance in the season to come. But what actually had happened at the solstice ritual two months before, when this top was used? Seth had spun the top, but unfortunately he had stuffed the holes with damp feathers, so when he spun the top, the feathers would not fly out. Seth was now afraid this meant there would be no whales. [Sure enough, in

June 1989 I heard by satellite telephone the distressing news that during that year the hunters did not catch a single whale. The weather and ice conditions made it impossible. So the spinning top spoke the truth, albeit an unlucky truth. I could see Iñupiat spirit understandings were as strong as ever.]

I said good-bye to Seth and bundled up again against the storm. My house was about two hundred yards through the village. Out in the blizzard I found that when I walked out of Seth's door I could reach the road okay. So I strove forward, trying to keep my feet despite the wind. I struggled to the top of a snow drift, then another, then turned the corner, looking for the firehouse with its large red front and high roof. That should be my landmark. I saw only the vaguest outlines, which gave me no clue. It was hard to see anything. Maybe the firehouse was there, maybe not. Now I walked against the wind, over many drifts, up and down, up and down, walking, climbing, walking. I hadn't been looking at anything; I couldn't look. At length I came to a wall in front of me. It was a long barrier, a very high, white snowbank with no gap in it at all. An attempt at a road lay along this side of it. I quailed at this barrier because it was much too high to climb or see over, even if I could see anything.

A house stood further up on the left. That might be a help. Was I for some reason on the lagoon side, beside the snow fence? I didn't even think how I could have made such a circle. The lagoon? The day before the bus had negotiated the wide angle out toward the lagoon where there were few houses—a lonely place. A new car—a recreation vehicle—was parked on the roadside. If it had been a truck, I would have concluded I was on the south road, but this car meant I could be anywhere. I shuffled by it, thinking that maybe I could find my way into town on the left beyond the house. There was nothing beyond. I came back to the car and felt really tired of this battle. What was I going to do? How much longer could I fight, a tiring person, sixty-eight years old. Why, I was weak. This frightened me, and I sidled to the car to stand on its lee side for a moment and get out of the hurricane of cold. I had heard it was two degrees. I'd have to try the house. Supposing no one was in, and it was locked? I'd have to go from house to house. . . . What house? . . . Stupid head on me. Peering and peering back down the way I had come, I saw at the end, between monstrous wallops of falling snow, an opening in the view for a second. I saw two arches, round-topped things . . . big, arched structures, vague in the blur, like a pair of the arches at the Rockefeller Center, or like the McDonald's

Golden Arches. It was a very puzzling sight in Ivakuk. Had there been some changes? There couldn't be a McDonald's in Ivakuk. *Arches?* I struggled forward for a better look. Ah. The arches were actually two circles. Of course. They were the satellite dishes for the telephone system. (When I tell this story, the Iñupiat storm with helpless laughter.) I looked at the nearby house again. Was it Velma's? It had four windows, so it was definitely not her tiny cottage. Still, I set off that way. I was probably on my own street; I had to be. But it was not Velma's, and I was still lost, with just the dishes to go by. So I went to them, my dishes, my English-invented radar dishes, past which I had often jogged. And as I approached the corner where they stood, it all became clear. The great ice barrier was along the south shore road, not the lagoon side. I was dangerously near nothing, near the waste of the wide beach and the ocean ice. At the foot of the satellite dishes I saw my usual turning that led away from the sea, with a huge drift across it, which I climbed gratefully, and then another drift, and there indeed was Velma's house. I was on the home stretch. Past Sam's house, past my own, which I couldn't approach directly because of a snowdrift, then on a few yards to find a gap in the drift, then back toward the door—and in to warmth and relief. It could have been otherwise.

All that day I heard calls from house to house on the Citizens Band. "No elders' lunch." "No bus." "No stove oil deliveries." "Planes canceled." One or two responsible Iñupiak women were running the village. Everything was latched down and secure. There was one woman at the school, one at the municipal office, one at the store. The electricity kept up. The telephone was dead. The Citizens Band was okay. Nobody knew anything about the clinic; they only knew about the power station.

Overnight I began to hear the backing-up sound of beeping from the snow movers, those great monsters with giant pans in front of them, with their headlights and rear lights on, and I hoped the drivers had a warm cabin while they worked all night on the clogged vital spots of the village. The Iñupiat were keeping the village alive. The next morning many huge drifts still remained to be worked on, though they had cleared the drifts in front of the store and the power station. Now came an announcement. "Elders lunch is on." There was no bus, but when I arrived, most of the elders were there, brought by their grown children on snowmobiles, thus illustrating the Iñupiat care for the elders. At lunch my satellite dish story went over just fine. The young cook poised to listen with a big spoon in her hand, her body thoughtful, a scene of beauty to madden a Van Gogh. Then the gale of laughter. We watched out of the window while the snow mover with its pan plunged hugely into the snowdrift outside, collecting tons of snow and retreating to dump them outside the village.

I completed my visits. The big drift by the community center had already been sliced in two, leaving a track deep into its heart and out the other side. I saw people come out of their homes and dart into their sheds, where they stored frozen meat and also kept their electric freezers—and back again with haunches of caribou or whole frozen fish. Many were living on subsistence food only and were doing fine. All were cheerful. One house had no electricity, one had a broken furnace and would grow cold, many who had telephones found them dead, and one house had its chimney blown down. A White man, who was inspector of housing, paid a call at my house. He spoke too loudly but was genial in a professional way. The Iñupiat inspector who accompanied him came from a distant village. He told us that his wife was pregnant and the baby was two weeks overdue. He himself had yet another village to inspect. He wanted *home*, poor guy.

On further visits I sometimes experienced spirit episodes like those I had already encountered. On one occasion I arrived in the summer. Once again I mounted the town bus at the airstrip to ride into the village. Once more we passed the dull two-mile stretch of gravel. Then as we turned the dogleg corner by the big machine shops, I realized strongly that I was back home again. I was on my way to Jim Agnasagga's. Various friends who happened to ride the bus in town said "Welcome home" to me with a grin.

On the first Sunday I entered the church. To begin with I sat in front with Gabe; then I realized I would not be able to count the people from that position, so I moved to my old seat in the second pew from the back on the left, where I used to sit with Joanna before she died. The church filled. A woman resembling Joanna sat down across the aisle. Immediately, I had the distinct feeling, triggered by the appearance of the other woman, that Joanna herself was beside me in the empty space in the pew. I was concerned about her upper arm as in the old days. She was palpably there, the beaky, tender, solemn woman with something like an impediment in her speech, clothed in the dark velveteen parka and crowned with the huge ruff—Joanna, whose eyes had seen the Easter apparition of her dead sister—brown, tottering Joanna, favoring one arm, keeping it zipped inside the body of the parka with just an empty sleeve outside, the upper arm bone riddled with cancer. I had a direct sense she was there. And I humbly accepted the sense. It persisted until Agatha, at the other end of the pew, glanced over without looking at me, her face puckered into a pout. It switched off my sense of Joanna like a light. Joanna was gone. When Agatha turned away from me again the memory of the sense came back but not the sense itself.

During these later visits to Ivakuk I lodged with Jim Agnasagga. Our conversations became important to him and me, and they were so near to the bone that I felt impelled to write them down. [As Dan Rose has said in an article entitled "Reversals," "The most radical position that we can take [as anthropologists], and take it we must, is to imagine the democracy of this new aesthetic space where poetic voices reach across to one another and where they contend and converse" (Rose 1991, 300).]

Jim Agnasagga was striding about in the living room with a sleeping baby on his shoulders. His hair was a little on end, and his eyebrows were lowered in thought. He was hesitant about how to put things into words.

"It's the animals. They know four times as much as we do. I want—I want there to be no pollution. What about the pollution at Gray Cat?" Gray Cat was an extremely productive lead and zinc mine situated in the region. "Fish are bottoming up on the river there. Next they'll bring in a road. I'm afraid. In ten years' time it'll all be changed here. If only we were on our own. It's good that we're Eskimos here, not Whites," he went on, shifting the position of the baby. "Our parents and grandparents, they faced changes. I go hunting; it's my life. And at the same time I'm head supervisor of the stone-crushing plant for the North Slope Borough road project." His eyebrows were raised.

As he spoke I envisioned Ivakuk Village, the ice, then the clock time world of Jim's job, and the clock itself as the point of variance between the two worlds. As if he knew my thoughts, he said, "This idea you have to have a goal: we 'must' do such and such a thing in a *set* time. You just need to forget all that and simply do it. It'll get done."

As Jim walked to and fro he was almost praying, speaking in the sad, reverent voice of the Native American.

"The elders," he said, thinking. "If only the young said to the elders, *'What would you want to say to us if we listened?'* The elders would have to tell them."

Jim and I saw things very much alike. I thought, "We liberal Whites have learned a considerable amount from American natives." Various cultural differences were churning inside Jim, and he was influencing me too.

In 1990 Jim's young sister died of cancer. Many people in the village had a suspicion that something at the site of an old nuclear bomb project might be the cause of this case and also of the other numerous fatalities in the village. I had been thinking of ways that a few politically conscious people might influence the authorities to look into the matter. But Jim had a different way in mind.

"What do you think? Can a few friends—" he bent toward me, "you know what I mean, *shamans*—succeed when most of the people aren't in it?"

"Oh yes indeed," I said, nodding. "I believe they could." I remembered how Jim had told me that it was the Ivakuk shamans who had taken Stalin off the face of this world.

Jim went on, "The trouble is, they compete. Each one tries to be the strongest." We thought for a time together. I knew about competing shamans.

"When there were three thousand of us here," he said, "they competed. Too many people."

I thought to myself, "Maybe yes, though not too many for the ecology. Perhaps too many—"

"Socially," broke in Jim. We were following each other's thoughts.

"Exactly."

He said: "I have made a commitment. I've opened myself to whatever comes." This was to shamanism. That was the way he put it. "Christianity is different. . . ."

He made these throw-away elliptical statements, hesitant, looking at me warm-eyed.

"There's a unity in an Eskimo village you don't get outside. Everyone cares. To catch a whale you need many people; that's it."

At this point a stranger entered the room and asked Jim on the side, "Who's she?"

"A blood relative," said Jim, grinning at me.

In 1992 Jim brought in a seal that was covered with a stiff, yellow stain. He laid it by his shed and didn't want to eat it. He told me that one in three seals were sinking these days when they were shot, not floating as usual.

"That's because they're skinny; there's not much fat on them. They're not getting enough to eat." Jim had been so worried he got in touch with the Environmental Protection Agency.

Later he told me something in a hesitating voice, "—I went to the hill—" He pointed toward the southern cape. Jim could hardly bring himself to say what he did there. He laughed deprecatingly. "And I *talked* to the seals in their own language. Oh boy, and I came home and fell very ill—I had a fever of 102 degrees. It came to the point when I couldn't breathe and I nearly died. . . . I knew it was connected. The animals were hurting me. Why?" He paused. "But I didn't die. Whatever. . . . The missing tom cod came back and the seals were fed."

Jim and I made up a list of what was needed in Ivakuk. These were the benefits Iñupiat dancing provided: healing, good weather, and the bringing of animals. The unity of the village was necessary for this, Jim said, the unity of young and old.

June 10, 1992, Wednesday. Jim told me of a curious experience he had had when he was on a trip from Prudhoe Bay to Atkasut, in North Slope oil country. He and two other Ivakuk men were driving a huge oil-drill vehicle through a strange region. "Eric and Dicky [the latter now dead by his own hand] and I were in the cab. Because of how the rig is, we could only travel between three and four miles an hour. The rig was for offshore drilling and testing of beach and landing conditions for oil wells." Jim made a gesture of shame. "I don't think that's a good thing. But it was my job, see?

"We had a breakdown for two days. Huh, a difficult trip. I was kind of guide and biologist on the trip, and I wanted to keep awake, though it wasn't my shift to drive the driller rig. I tried, I tried to keep awake. But I went to sleep. Then I woke up. Inside the cab were Frankie, the dead harpooner, Sid [now also dead from suicide], and a whole lot of living Ivakuk people, friends of mine. I was very puzzled. I said, 'There are a whole lot of people in this cab'—and went to sleep again. I woke again and the same thing happened the second time. I said, 'There are a *whole lot of people* in this cab.' Okay, the time came for my shift to drive, and then Eric slept. *He* woke up and said, 'There are a whole lot of people in this cab.' I never found out exactly who the others were. I had an idea two of them were White. This happened to Eric twice, just as it had happened to me. Then it was Eric's turn to drive, and Dicky slept, and he woke, and the same thing happened with him, twice.

"When we arrived, and we were sitting down over coffee and doughnuts, it occurred to us that we'd all had the same experience. It's that place; it's always like that: people get lost, lanterns are seen beckoning travelers, and if they go toward them they never come back, and so on."

I could picture the rig with the haunted cabin riding slowly across the night, and Jim's puzzlement.

"Dreams are funny," I said, and told him my dream of the man carrying broken glass and what happened afterward, and the other odd things that happened to me.

"*I know,*" said Jim.

He kept showing an interest in shamanism, evidence of a gift of his own. I mentioned the caribou man. Jim turned round full face to me.

"Do you believe in Caribou Man?" he asked me, squinching his eyes with great seriousness.

"To tell you the truth I think I do," I said.

"Good," he said, greatly relieved. "My friend always told me, 'Look at the feet; you see the caribou feet. There are strangers in town? You don't know who they are? Look at the feet.'

"It's that grave," he went on, referring to the cause of the restless spirit.

"There's a body in it?"

"I haven't been down there for a long time," said Jim. "I heard the coffin was protruding. You know what, they should bury 'em away from the overhang. The shamans used to say, never go under an overhang, it will descend on you. Maybe it's one chance in a hundred, but that will be it. You shouldn't go under an overhang. The shamans are offended. People don't remember their advice."

June 12, 1992, Friday. Several of us were seated around Jim's table, drinking tea and chewing muktuk. One of the company had just come in from the borough. We were haunted by visions of death: the recent suicide of Dicky, Suellen's son, for instance; the wife coming in and seeing Dicky's face mashed by the bullet he put under his chin, with the baby right there on his lap. The borough woman began to describe the year's events in her home town, speaking very seriously.

"Two men were lost on the ice last winter. Two. Now two whales were caught this spring. Two. Okay. Then you heard about the two women? When the people pulled in the second whale—it was a big one sixty feet long—the tackle broke. The hawser flew back and struck one woman and exposed her brains. She died immediately. The arm of the other woman was torn off in front of the whole crowd. She was a Peruvian. She died in the hospital later. Another was medevacked out and recovered. Two women died. Now listen to this. The bones of two men became exposed in graves by the overhang in Barrow. Two men. The bones were put in a box and kept in my office."

All were silent.

"Those dead are angry." she said. "They ought to be buried with a preacher in graves well inland. We should have government-cleared equipment to do it." She leaned back.

"What about the toggle head? In the whale?" I asked.

"Yes. When they cut up that whale they found inside it one of those old Eskimo toggle heads that haven't been used for a hundred years. An ivory one with a stone blade in it, the sort that goes on the top of a harpoon. They reckon that whale was at least a hundred years old."

"So it's true," I said. The report was going around everywhere.

What did it all mean? The people were reading the events much as a Pentecostal elder "discerns" the meaning of what is said during speaking in tongues. There was some meaning, and Jim thought so too. One thing was clear: the message of the dead was being given emphatically, even with violence.

Jim returned to the subject of the coffin at Ivakuk. "Things have changed here," he said. "Our people who knew about such things always used to go down to the point if they needed a north wind or whatever. They went to the place of the spirits at the point." I knew that place. "Our people could talk to the spirits. But now, with the grave exposed, the spirits are angry."

This circle at the table was a circle of real friends. This could not be just fieldwork for me, yet of course it could not help being that. Many anthropologists find that fieldwork relationships turn into real relationships. Is it true that when they do not, that is, when the relationship remains not "real," it should kept going for the sake of scientific research? This is one problem, that of "real" scientific research involving "nonreal" or superficial relationships. Then there is the curious fact that shared spirit experiences often bring into existence real relationships; in other words, what is supposed to be not real creates what is real.

And then, what does one find going on? Filaments and sequences of thinking the same thoughts; prophetic dreams; odd effects of healing; sensing the dead. ▪

I was skinning a seal with Annie again. This was a natchiq, a small spotted seal. As usual, she was taking off the skin, and I took off the fat, cutting chunks and slivers and putting them into a bucket, where they would drain and produce seal oil naturally when kept in the kitchen and turned every day. Seal oil contains seventeen vitamins, is a tasty condiment, and makes an excellent medication for bronchitis and chest ailments.

We worked on the body of the seal. The dainty limbs, the hands and the legs, were clothed in delicate plush. The face lay tilted back with a spirit in it, giving itself, telling me directly of its self-sacrifice; the eyes did not see now, but the soul inside spoke to me each time I looked.

"Seal, I heard you," I said. My eyes caressed its little fulfilled head with the happy whiskers.

No doubt I "heard" in a White person's way, somewhat different from the way of the Iñupiat, to whom the animals mean survival itself. But there was a connection.

During the days of the midnight sun, Naluq's family does not go to bed until 1:30 A.M., though I am always in bed at 12. When they finally assemble, I hear a chorus of cheerful voices weaving into each other, along with musical threats and cajolements from the voice of their mother, Naluq, deeper and fuller than the children's. I hear the voices from my bed, free voices with no attempt at politeness—there's an outburst of coughing from the seven-year-old boy. Baleful and musical voices, each confident, one along with the other, each voice fully keyed, free, varying, many-colored. Again comes the baleful, careworn threat from the mother. The boy forgets to cough. The baby's continual noise, a confident imitation of the sound of the voices, only without the words, is withdrawn. The mother's voice suddenly sharpens into a lightning bolt of warning, then falls away. And as soon as she speaks, the seven-year-old coughs, a voice from a lower level driven by no thought. Now the baby's *"Eah! Eah!"* comes in again at that lower level, but laden with thought of a kind. I am hearing Native American voices speaking in English with their own intonation. Up comes a puzzled question, whose tone is set to rise throughout the sentence and wave with defiant dissatisfaction at the end. The mother's answer-

ing remarks in the dark register, rising and falling imperceptibly—
just calculated to penetrate as the words progress—manifest themselves somehow as sorrow.

Her last utterances before they all fall asleep at 1:30 A.M. in
broad daylight have leveled to a single tone, deep tuned, soft, and
full, on one note except for the gentle discontinuities that words
impart to a single note. Even further within that tone I hear plainly
the human, conscious, unmistakable message of tenderness. Finally,
from the depths of the house, from the couch in the living room,
comes up a strange, curled, male sound, the father speaking out of
a dream: one curled sound, then a helpless *"Harumph."* Jim's
voice.

After that there is nothing but the cough, cough, cough of the
five-year old girl.

Conclusion

Threads of Connectedness

Jim Agnasagga said, "About eleven years ago a case came up in the papers about a person who was cured by a tribal doctor. The newspaper's line was that this wasn't so and couldn't be so." Jim was sorrowfully indignant about it and turned to face me.

"You've got to tell it how it is, Edie. Tell them about tribal healing."

Ordinary life in Ivakuk is deeply involved with spirit experience. The ability to have these experiences is like the use of a faculty, eyesight for instance, something one uses continually. Life would be very strange without it. The recurring cases in my narrative are all of much the same cloth. Even the near-death experience appears to be all of a piece with the shaman's four-day episode.

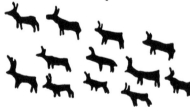

It seems that with care one can develop a listening posture to these events and learn to discern them, just as Claire discerned her patients' troubles and the Assembly of God members discerned what their fellow members meant when they spoke in tongues. Similarly, one comes to know with that different kind of knowledge that, for instance (a) something does pass when one heals a person, (b) singing, dancing, and drumming are not just art forms, but bring the animals, and (c) in-tune persons and the weather are not unconnected.

But how do these miracle-like events come about? There seem to be definite and discernible outlets, passages opened by the songs, paths for the soul.

Everyone was interlinked in Ivakuk, in kinship interrelationships that produced an effect like a well-made jigsaw puzzle: if one lifts up one corner of it, the whole puzzle comes with it.[1] Nevertheless, this characteristic was not merely rooted in the balances and counterbalances of the interwoven kinship system, but was more fundamentally rooted in a sense that that social interweaving did indeed have its role in nourishing: that is, that same sense that made possible the conversation of bodies in healing, the communication with the food animals, the dreams, the warnings, and the visions that constituted communication with spirits.

Thus, I place the state of connectedness as the milieu that spirits and their activity foster and, having provided that milieu, they can grow in it—a circular process. "The whale wants us to become spirit conscious, so it gives itself to us. Then it can reincarnate, and we can too." I have had to look beyond the old rules of causality—even those of psychology or social conditioning—to see the hole in the continuum of positivist causality and see human causation as often located beyond, in the spirit world, as Clem and the others saw it.

There existed a network of these experiences, with many threads. In my education in Ivakuk I was encouraged (mainly by Clem) to follow the connectedness of the hunter with the animal, principally in the drumming, which "brings the caribou." It was early on in my fieldwork when I heard about whale reincarnation; the whale's spirit did not die when the men caught it, but it reincarnated, refleshed its body to make a new whale. Through the same hole in the continuum, as it were, connected to reincarnation, clock time was nullified. For instance, this showed at the Halfway Place in the Whaling Festival. Time was spiked by the flagpole that linked the ancient whale skull to the present-day boat on its pedestal of celebration, thus bringing a future reincarnated whale. The confounding of time also took place somewhere between the prophetic dreams and their fulfillment, and in Seth's divination by means of his spinning top, predicting the absence of whales. Somehow, in contact with spirit things one's dreams jumped time. In the spirit mode the spirit body knows no barriers of space (the Qusaqsuna case), no barriers of time. In 1990 a small boy in Ivakuk told his mother, "I'm going to die tomorrow." The next day a bus backed into him and he was killed. The village was appalled, at the same time marveling at the child's premonition. Time could fold back.

When such a thing happened, it was in some circumstance of importance—there was something definite to learn. The impact at these times was that of absolute certainty, "apodicticity," to use a term of Husserl's (quoted from Laughlin 1994).

In addition, randomness came to be celebrated, connected with the undifferentiated generosity of nature, the hunter's life, and also divination, and shown in the throwing gestures, the scattering of candy, even the blanket toss—celebrations of nonlogic and chance. Even bingo had that quality. These phenomena constituted another path, a thread that also became part of the network (that further continuum) of experience.

So a major thread ran this way: spirit communication plus the conversation of bodies, plus communication with the food animals, together maintained the skilled ability to connect subtly and deeply, so that subsistence remained in the milieu of connectedness, language reflected connectedness, history continued to firmly keep it in honor, and the complex and interwoven kinship system could rest permanently in connection. From these branched out the awareness of reincarnation, the nonprimacy of clock time, prophetic dreams, divination, and the celebration of chance.

Another thread, also deriving from spirit communication and the spirit work of the animals, connected with the progression of the cosmological cycle, understood by the Iñupiat as the ever ongoing process of birth, food, death, and rebirth, with spirit kinetics driving it. A living spirit looked out at me from Kaglik's dead bone masks—from bone, the bottom line of death. Also I strongly sensed the spirit in the head of the whale and in Joanna, dead but back on the church pew, here repeating Joanna's vision of her sister Paula. Here also one may understand the soul trying to leave and go to the jade floor of heaven and, with grand nonlogic, also to come to rest in a newborn baby—which connects with the healing shaman who could sense the soul leaving the body and its whereabouts. The shaman herself or himself, many times in her or his lifetime, was taken over by her destiny as a healer. She was taken and blanked out in those episodes, horribly aware of the aggressive side of the spirit that afflicted her. So she came to terms. She was not her own property but was a natural element in the communal whole. She found that she would not have it otherwise. "She has God's hands." "She has the Blessing."

The threads that led to the animal spirits revealed the whale spirit and the eagle spirit as the dominant, self-sacrificial spirits for all Iñupiat. Animal guardians were slightly different: the polar bears that visited Netta and young Kehuq, for example. A corpus of narratives are told about "a certain orphan" who was terrorized by a small animal called a *kikituq*, somewhat like a marten or wolverine, with legs that spread wide from its body, extremely strong. (This animal is not to be found in any list of fauna but finds a place in the spirit animal category.) The orphan finally discovered how to use the animal. It should be tucked into the sleeve of one's parka, cosied and nursed, and then allowed to peek out. Then it would be friendly. When its owner was hunting, it would emerge from his sleeve and point in the direction of the caribou, thereby bringing the caribou to the hunter's gun. This kind of transformation, from aggressiveness to helpfulness, tallied with much of the tribal experience of acquiring an animal helper—a being that started as a savage spirit.

As for the whale and the eagle, these spirit beings achieved reincarnation—the regrowing of the parka—and their doings were told in the whale and the eagle protohistories. Parallel with these, reports of human reincarnation were common in Ivakuk. About half the kindergarten class of 1992 were named after some tragically dead person of the village. Naming was consciously done with an ear to the spirit that might want to be reborn in the new child—a kind of divinatory sense (compare Fienup-Riordan 1983,157; Søby 1990). This was specially so in the case of twins: when one died, the other took the spirit of the dead one. Reincarnation was considered positively desirable, as with Native Americans generally. The soul, especially one whose passing was violent, was welcomed back into the family for a better go-around next time. This is unlike the philosophy behind South Asian reincarnation, according to which the ideal outcome is to go upward to Nirvana or to heaven with the gods, and not to be reincarnated at all (Obeyesekere, forthcoming).

We may in a shadowy way, then, identify a "soul" that can slip from one body to another. It is not exactly the same as the soul that slips out of a person when she or he dies, though the point is arguable.

As for the associated craft of healing, various spirit ideas were concerned. I myself was learning the techniques in a very elementary way. One could not stay on this side of medical beliefs for such healing. One had to begin to see illness as some kind of substance—then the healing worked. It did seem to work. Thus, the illness appeared to be a kind of spirit stuff, offending inside the body of the sufferer, telling lies to the afflicted and infecting her—not only with those germs seen under a microscope, but with spirit germs in a sense, quite palpable. There were useful ways to get rid of such bad intrusions—by means of bodily treatment by the healers and by soul retrieval.

The ideas about the experience of the spirit near death and at death, leaving for another world, ran back into the experience of the shaman Qusaqsuna when his spirit left on a journey to his home—the spirit journey—also into the experience of the whale's nature and whale reincarnation, also human reincarnation, also the soul's state—even absence—in the body's illness, and the ghost's visitations after death. All were related to all. The adventures of such soul entities have been depicted in various masks of Eskimo art—with their soul doors; soul rings or hoops, which are the universes; visionary ivory eyes; and the like (Fienup-Riordan 1990, 49–67). Of course, souls have been depicted in our culture as floating figures, by William Blake, Gustave Dore, lately by Gould Hulse (who has not yet published his pictures), and many others. I contend that many of these were, like the Eskimo ones, depictions of experience. Visible soul manifestations do occur, and they are very mixed in meaning. Records exist of a wide variety of imponderable beings.

In the Protestant church at Ivakuk, Protestant prayer was mingled with visions experienced by the people. The visions contained a poetic and emotional dimension, from the impact of being bodily and literally felt. Annie's vision of the water of life, her mouth hanging open, receiving it, was sensed by her as concrete reality.

The Problem of Spirit Action. The experience of absolute certainty has been termed by Charles Laughlin (1994, 115, quoting Husserl) "apodicticity," derived from *apo-* "beyond, separate from" and *-dicticity* "speech." "I can't put it into words," was a frequent saying of Claire's, and as I have shown, sometimes others had trouble relating their experiences. Apodicticity deals basically with perceptions—perceptions tagged with a special quality, as experienced by mystics, meditators, and visionaries. Apodicticity well describes Inupiat spirit perception. Then what about the nonordinary *actions,* the work, not just perception of the spirit? These are exemplified by Claire in her healing, Robert with his life-saving rope, and Qusaqsuna's journey. The term *psychokinesis* and the strongly held theories of spiritualists, with their "astral bodies," or "energy" and "vibration" certainties, are too particularized, tightly held, and often inflexible to meet the real sense of the acts of Claire and the others. How are we to go about finding a lightweight, pervious, adjustable theory to make some sense of the abilities of the Iñupiat? It does no harm to use what the Iñupiat themselves say, as recorded in this book. This is narrow in one sense, in that the Iñupiat would not include the Hindu chakra system, for instance, in their thinking. But in another sense there is a greater certainty that the Iñupiat system is practical and not allied to an elaborate religious theology that would render it inflexible and impervious. It more closely resembles the way traditional African doctors carry out their treatments—by rule of thumb—that is, "if they work." This is how the African doctors are making ground, gradually improving their treatments. Many of the successes of these and Iñupiat practitioners come about because both allow themselves to be guided by their own spirit tutelaries, whether this spirit is Jesus or an ancestor spirit. The spirit's guidance is what matters to these healers, not whether they are theologically or theoretically correct.

It is in the ambience of this freedom, then, this care to do the actual experiencing, this closeness to the body—that flashes occur—for instance, the sense of the trouble coming out. I referred earlier to flashes in the whale-hunting milieu, and in healing it is the same. So much for where and when they happen. But why? And what exactly is happening?

It is a very intimate thing, very much concerned with the human body. One can develop the sense; one can see the presence or the absence of a soul in a person or a body. Then, being aware of a person's soul, one wants to learn more. Having one's hands on a person's sick tissues and really wanting to help, one can sense the unhappiness of the tissues. It is easier when wanting to help someone else. This happens to be a fairly fool-proof rule—it is easier when wanting to help someone. This was probably the case long before Christianity and the people of the book. It is a characteristic that has something to do with the collective, the life in "connectedness." Among the Iñupiat the quality of connectedness provides a milieu that easily feeds healing, life-saving acts, altering the weather, and so on.

We are dealing with elusive imponderables here. Not many natives on the North Slope liked strict categories and definitions. A spirit's existence (say, a polar bear helper) was felt to be absolute when the experience was in progress. That is, when there was an occasion in which the people were reporting one manifestation, the other types were absent and were then not a matter of concern. Theologies or systems of spirits were not a preoccupation, nor was this due to a low level of intellectualization, but it was in keeping with the very nature of the subject matter.

As I have described it, spirit perception and spirit experience came in flashes during the vicarious events of the year. This "flash" characteristic shows the elusiveness of the subject matter and teaches the need for the utmost caution in the matter of ethnographic documentation. No dogmatic statements can be made. My words should not be taken in that sense, for like most fieldworkers I was feeling my way. Just as the Iñupiat had been doing since they began, I too needed to keep an open mind in order to learn.

There was a strong connection among the people in Ivakuk on the basis of the "now"—an intricate "circulation-of-the-blood" of their learning, as it were. The Iñupiat ears were alerted by one case after another, and these cases all led together into that peculiar form of spirit consciousness that I saw in the 1980s and 1990s, inextricably mixed with Christianity and only operating in an on-the-spot manner, contextually. And it must have been in the same on-the-spot manner that these cases led them in ages past, before Christianity, to work with the variations in spirit concepts. The Iñupiat were used to the flashes they received. Nevertheless, they still marveled at each one. They certainly did, for example, during the buzz of excitement in the village at the appearance of Satan, alias the drunken master of the ancient science, grown huge in form and in a bad temper. This was also called a "ghosting" in the village; at the time it represented one clear form of spirit manifestation.

Thus, in the process of weaving realities—weaving the social flavor and the body together—I struggled to deal with some very difficult material. The spirit forms were quite clear when one encountered them, but would in a sense fade and crack if forced into strict categories. It is enough to say that, in spite of the sparsity of linguistic distinctions (only "soul," "spirit," and "ghost" were much in use), spirit awareness was as alive as ever in Ivakuk, operating as a kind of periodic flash charge of the culture.

Spirit processes thrummed through the village constantly, in every vein and artery of its working. Many people, not only Claire, had experiences that they could not possibly doubt, apodictic experiences, those of absolute certainty. Annie had them often, and not only she, but Sam, Robert, Jim, Clem, Netta, Joanna, Kaglik, Dionne, Madeline, Stella, young Kehuq, young Louis, young Peter, the young girl Marilyn, old Michael, Uncle Runiq, Aunt Judy, old Kehuq, Qusaqsuna—being individuals with whom I was familiar, and there were certainly others. For many of them the experiences came in the form of spirit perception, but with Claire,

Suellen, Robert, Clem, Netta, Uncle Runiq, Aunt Judy, old Kehuq, and Qusaqsuna it was a matter of spirit action: healing or shamanic deeds of power or lifesaving. My own most vivid experience in Ivakuk was the time when I was conscious that Joanna was beside me, after her death.

The problems of analysis regarding this material are not likely to go away. Should we still study such events as socially derived "symbolism," or alternatively as counters in a game of political differences? Or should we treat them as traditional givens, and leave it at that? It is possible, though, to regard them as events in their own right, needing a particular kind of effort to reach understanding, as phenomena to be recognized as a permanent feature of this ecological world. A field of study is beginning to develop in the anthropology of consciousness and the anthropology of religion, in which researchers do experience what their field people experience. They take their experiences seriously and record them in the spirit of the natural historian. I have used Michael Jackson's argument from his book *Paths toward a Clearing: Radical Empiricism and Ethnographic Inquiry* (1989) to maintain, like him, that ritual experience proves itself to be true and valid *in use,* not as a preordained system or structure. In exactly this way, the Iñupiat's spirit-related life has validity in use. Ritual is a matter of process; symbols live when in use. Categories of spirits have of course been described before. Merkur (1985, 225–46) has described them for early Canadian Inuit culture. He refers to *iñua* "person" or "soul"; *tornaq* "spirit helper"; the breath-soul that finishes at death and lacks mind: the name-soul that is reincarnated; the free soul that goes out on a shaman journey; the ghost; and wind indwellers, constituting a universal breath-soul. Among the Iñupiat, ideas about spirits appear to have changed as the decades passed, as the emphasis on a given category of spirit changed or faded. But if the occasion arose and events concerning certain spirits came to the fore, then that category would stand out in full dimension and be well sensed and appreciated.

In Ivakuk this happened in many cases: Joanna's spirit, for one; the Jackson family's polar bear spirit; reincarnated spirits like Sam Junior's spirit, which left him after his suicide and entered a new baby who was born with a mark on his neck at the place where the bullet had entered Sam Junior's neck; the spirits of the huge beasts, the whales. And so on. There existed in the Iñupiat this massive other sense, a sense arising and developing in response to the spirits that that faculty began to sense. The spirits were out there, not in the people's heads.

A kind of natural history of all this lies ready for the taking. For me it was necessary to show its workings in the context of the year's events, just as the events befell, in order to show their living nature.

Again, *what exactly is a spirit?* A reverberation emanating in its old milieu from some strong personality that once was around? If spirits are reverberations, why are they so strong and full of intentions? We may have to come to terms with the fact that we are not the only souls occupying this earth, that there are indeed other entities, and that the sense needed to communicate with them requires a little care to develop. We have developed faculties before. Speech and reading, from the beginning, needed care, to be sure. We exercised that care and patience gladly. Now we find there is a continuum of such possibilities, and we have the chance to learn some of them in our own time. This one constitutes a sense—hesitant, like the way Jim Agnasagga tries to say it; all one can say is that it is very nearly beyond words—if the words are at all superficial. Put one's hands in it, and it flows off like water. But the hands feel it.

Notes

Introduction

1. *Iñupiat* is the plural and adjectival form of the singular form, *Iñupiaq,* meaning "original inhabitant" or a member of the northern Alaskan Eskimo people. The dual form, for two persons, is *Iñupiak.*

2. *Ivakuk* means "searching for an animal." I have changed the names of places and persons to protect the right to privacy of the individuals concerned. It is much to be regretted that, for that reason, I cannot give bibliographical references for publications that directly describe "Ivakuk" village.

3. For general ethnography on the region, see Rasmussen (1952), Oquilluk (1981), Lantis (1947), Chance (1966), Spencer (1959), Burch (1975), Iñupiat Community of the Arctic Slope (1979), and Blackman (1989), among many others. The scholarship is rich. The anthropological approach has varied among straight ethnography, some psychological analysis, occasional structural analysis, fine transcriptions of native accounts and stories—sometimes even achieving poetry—and descriptions of economic conditions.

4. In February 1993 I joined the elected heads of the village and the borough in their protest at the United Nations and at the U.S. Department of Energy.

5. For regional publications on healers see Lucier, VanStone, and Keats (1971), Juul (1979), and King (1962), among many others who have done valuable work on tribal doctors and shamanism.

6. Iñupiat accounts tell of a man who actually turned into a whale. Detailed Iñupiat accounts of the spirits who lived underground at the end of the beach and possessed the power to change the wind and the weather have been recorded.

7. Ethnographers in other fields have done similar work, such as Trawick among the Tamil (1990), Lavie among the Bedouin (1990), Kondo in Japan (1990), Karen McCarthy Brown with Voudou practitioners (1991), and Abu-Lughod in the Western Desert of Egypt (1993).

8. Mathematicians have experimented with totally random systems,

such as the turbulence of water in a pipe, drops falling inconsistently from a tap, traffic snarls, population swings among wild herds, and the weather, and have accumulated their vagaries, plotting them on a graph. That process, astonishingly, produces a curious double whorl—two close and connected cocoons, known as the strange attractor (Gleick 1987).

2: A Dream of the Loss of Childhood

1. Owing to pressure from the Alaska Federation of Natives and native communities under the Indian Reorganization Act, a new federal law was passed in 1989, extending the time limit for the protection of Iñupiat and other native lands from alienation. The original protection lasted only until 1991. I arrived in Ivakuk at an uneasy time, 1987.

2. Netta's account of the eagle was the first of many accounts I encountered during the following seven years about the tingmiaqpak, the shamanic eagle. The corpus of narratives constitutes one of the great origin epics of the northern native world. More details are given in chapter 9.

3: The Healer

1. The telephone was a conch shell that Philip put to his ear. A cord led from it into his doctor's black bag, in which he stored amulets and herbal medicines. I took down his words in his trance, being the verbalized messages he was receiving from the distant copper-mining town of Ndola (E. Turner 1986).

2. In November I worked out an arrangement with Claire for language instruction. We had many useful sessions. I did not organize formal healing instruction because this instruction was best given when cases occurred.

4: Embattled Politics

1. Much later, from 1993 onward, Micky Hoffman skillfully implemented the rights of the IRA to take over and actually buy all the Ivakuk land, including the back country, forming first the Ivakuk Land Department and then the Native Village of Ivakuk; afterward the Native Village began claims to the control of public security, the school, business, and gradually everything under the state and municipal governments—in other words, native sovereignty, the hope of every Alaskan native. I saw his moves as part of a very clever chess game, first protecting his king by castling and then making further gambits.

5: The Taste of Sea Mammal

1. Some might term Clem's type of history *myth*. I have been asked by Iñupiat not to use terms like *legend* and *story* in my writings, but to use the term *protohistory*. Some readers may feel I am promoting the Iñupiat's

way of life and disvaluing science or non-Iñupiat religions. The Iñupiat would say that theirs is only one of the many ways. Velma Tukumavik said to me, admonishing me for my anger against the Whites, "We don't want to make Whites suffer in revenge for the suffering they have given us." I claim no exclusive rights for the Iñupiat and their spirit gifts, but they must retain the right to their own way of life.

Geertz humorously claims, in his relativist anthropology, that "to be human is to be Javanese," as it were—or Iñupiat, or whatever particularities work (personal communication). By the same rule we can recognize how each people's religion works for them. The culture of Ivakuk constitutes a single web that informs most of the things they do, apart from the workings of the American school in the village and apart from other outside influences. The school is in the business of ripping the web away as rubbish. The value of the web has not yet been recognized.

2. In Mexican Indian history there arose a similar consciousness of the four races, colored according to the North American Indian basic colors, and this took expression in a statue showing persons of the four races, red, white, yellow, and black, facing in the four directions. The statue used to stand in the center of the atrium of the basilica of Our Lady of Guadalupe at Mexico City, the most heavily attended shrine of folk Christianity in the Americas.

7: Winter

1. The direction or valency of these acts seems to differ from that of the world of commoditization, in which we spend most of our time and from which we apparently have no escape (Mauss 1954). Recently anthropologists have drawn attention to the frequent merging of economic commodity exchange and gift exchange—either in the form of humanistic commodity exchange or as the corruption of gift exchange into a power ploy.

The prototype for the Iñupiat ritual act may be the generosity of wild nature, which overproduces without calculating any comeback. For the Iñupiat, a hunter-gatherer people, their gifting has less meaning when viewed as the struggle of all against all in a power structure than it does as a component of the idea of "cosmological cycling" that dominates the cosmologies of northern peoples—other components being reincarnation, spirit experience, and the connectedness that characterizes Iñupiat society generally. These are the meanings to which the people themselves respond, and about which they are articulate.

2. Ann Fienup-Riordan (1990, 45; 1994, 266–98) described the Yup'ik Eskimo bladder festival, held in late November, in which the bladders of seals that had been caught used to be hung up and feasted. At the end the bladders were taken down and pushed through a hole in the ice, so that the souls of the animals might be born again.

3. The cheer was a cheer of recognition. This was the celebration of

the old Iñupiat polyandry: the woman captain, who was the main organizer and recruiter for the whale hunt—although she rarely entered a canoe—used to link her crewmen together in a fervent loyalty, that of shared sex, polyandry. The persons concerned were her husband (the whaling captain) and the harpooner if he was not a blood relative. While hunting whales, the relationship between these two men had to be well bonded. It was curious that our supposed jealousy reaction did not operate, but instead there was bonding. The system of property rights that obtains in the West, the system that is the principal source of male authority over women, was almost nonexistent here, whereas the people's very survival depended on the alliance of males in the umiak boat, not their competition. Moreover, if one of the males lost his life, the widow was then not fully a widow but already had other stable relationships. Christianity has long since stopped the practice of polyandry on the North Slope.

4. The phenomenon of the nonsetting of the moon occurs only once every eighteen years and only in arctic or antarctic regions. I chanced to be in Ivakuk in the winter of 1987 to 1988, the year that this occurred (see Saladin-d'Anglure 1990).

8: Winter Solstice

1. It is possible that the so-called "arctic hysteria" (Foulks 1972), a madness that seized Eskimos during the dark winter months, causing them to run far out on the ice and act in a crazy manner, was the beginning stage of incipient shamanism, as described in chapter 18. Or what Foulks described may have been the result of repressed shamanism at the period of the most powerful White influence. At all events, it was not a simple pathology.

9: The Messenger Feast

1. In later years a competition between villages became more pronounced.

2. The drum of Kivgiq, the musical instrument itself, was unusual. It was shaped like a tall, square box. At first I speculated that the performers might have made use of Dorothy Ray and Alfred Blaker's 1967 illustrated book of Eskimo masks containing a picture of this box drum. Had they copied it? No. It turned out that performances had been taking place from time to time throughout the era during which the Kivgiq was forbidden. A "simulated" performance was given in one village in the late 1950s, which was the basis for the present one. In Ivakuk, Agatha Kuper remembered a Kivgiq festival in 1938 that was held in the mission hall and run by the parents of Tookruq, the dancing elder of chapter 5. Although much detail has survived from these old performers, much has undoubtedly been lost.

3. Baleen plates are the sifting plates possessed by all the baleen

whales. (The bowhead is the only whale the Iñupiat hunt.) These whales feed on tiny krill and plankton, sifting the sea water by means of a series of flexible, hairy plates set close together in the mouth, black in color. The material is also known as whalebone.

4. Geordie Tukumavik showed me how they played string puppets in a 1990 performance in Ivakuk, using a puppet animal traveling across the room from one wall to the other. Geordie's demonstration made the animal seem so alive that the effect was very strange.

5. The comic interlude is an ancient feature of ritual performance, found not only in early Italian opera but in Indian Kathakali temple theater, in Japanese Noh theater, and even in African funerals. René Devisch (1993, 45) explains that such interludes "bring people to relate to one another in the setting of specific experience and make them receptive for a new message or a transformation."

6. Research is presently being conducted by Justine Owens at the Behavioral Medicine and Psychiatry Department at the University of Virginia. She is collecting statistics and comparing experiences of those who have had near-death experiences, with attention to whether or not they were in life-threatening circumstances and whether or not they experienced healing or became healers later on.

7. Annie's experience was one of absolute certainty (see Laughlin 1994 on apodicticity, a term in phenomenology whose meaning includes the sense of conviction that comes with a religious experience).

11: The Grandmother Speaks a *Word*

1. Spencer (1959, 306–27) gives descriptions of various kinds of trance. One was the kind that Netta had just enacted, and another was the drumming and dancing performance. Spencer also describes how sorcerers might use their powers to pierce their enemies with small spear points, causing illness that would required the services of a healing shaman to extract the points. Netta's *word,* as distinct from her singing trance, was yet another type of shamanic action.

12: The Laughing Mask

1. At the time of Netta's near-death experience, her husband, Kehuq, was a well man and was running the post office. He was a great Iñupiat savant at that time, but when I knew him he was suffering from Alzheimer's disease.

2. Some scholars have written overviews of customs concerning shamans and healers (see for example Winkelman 1992). These are not intended to provide detailed pictures of the phenomena nested in their particular contexts. Clearly, no mapping out of features could ever substitute for the living experience itself. Many experiences have been so strong that, within the

societies concerned, entire culture-bound theologies have been erected on their basis, and conversely, the style of the culture colored each theology.

15: The Whale's Head

1. Clem revered his old culture. He was not a nationalist at that time because he did not have a political plank. Nor was he ready to put his people on a pedestal. But he saw through the hunger of many of the villagers for things American, for assimilation. He and a few others did much to maintain the old religion, which Christians were not supposed to call religion; and he tried to live its heritage of acts, its spirit acts—a phrase with a different meaning from *ritual*. Annie had her arm acting *for* her—she did not make the gesture. A healer appears to put out her hands into the spirit zone of the sick person and to let her hands act within it.

2. In Iñupiat society the product of any first achievement is given away, whether it is the first taking of a whale by a man, the first taking of a seal by a boy, or the first fashioning of bead earrings by a girl. This custom signals the immediate communalization of a newly developed ability—that is to say, the ability itself is now communally owned; and the giving away of the whole product is an acknowledgment of the social and maybe spirit origin of the ability. Also the giving away constitutes a naturally occasioned initiation of the person as a new producer for the community. Thus, the first catch or the first achievement becomes an occasion to celebrate the young person's majority, both among the Iñupiat and among the Yup'iit, the central Alaskan Eskimos (Fienup-Riordan 1990, 39–41). Such an initiation differs from socially performed initiations based on sexual maturity and marked by tests and ordeals, as found in Africa, but it may have some affinities with the American Indian vision quest, in which, after the young person has waited for four days in the wilderness, an animal spirit helper approaches the youth and becomes his or her guardian. The vision quest initiation requires the same kind of hunter's patience as is practiced among the Iñupiat.

3. The whales were now offering themselves to the village. Ivakuk caught five in all, the full quota, in spite of Matthew's failure with the bomb. This was because Robert and Clem both caught whales at the same time at the end of the migration period and were unaware that the other one was hunting. So they were not breaking the regulations.

4. Margie's slow step was considered by the people to be the slow movement of the whale. Indeed, analysts have argued that the woman "is" the whale. This would be more than "communication"; it would be identity. Such merging of symbolism into identity is a phenomenon that we may recognize as a particular mode of ritual understanding. Instead of Roy Wagner's "symbols that stand for themselves" (1986), we have obviated symbolism altogether. The notion that the woman *is* the whale is shown in another rite once frequently performed and still sometimes referred to—

the "harpooning" of the whaling captain's wife. The wife is the first to reach the edge of the ice when the season begins. Then she lies down on the ice with her legs toward the water. The men, who have been following her with the boat on a sled, now launch it, paddle out a little, then come toward her. The captain makes a ritual stab at her with his harpoon, without hurting her. She rises and starts walking back toward the village. (During her walk she is sometimes seen with a whale's tail emerging out of her mouth in a shamanic state of unity with the whale.) Simultaneously a whale rises in the water, and at once the waiting men intercept it with their boat and catch it. Here woman and whale are one, and that one is a shaman. Some masks are still carved showing a woman's face with the whale's tail emerging from her mouth.

5. In 1992 at the borough center, an accident occurred while a large whale was being hauled in. The cable broke, spun back, and killed two women who were helping to haul.

6. There were other references to the whale as a reincarnating, conscious, and all-knowing being. Commenting on a whale's vertebra carved by Kaglik into the shape of a human face, Clem said, "The face is the whale's face. It is different. When the whale's parka is taken off you see the whale's face. All animals have that. When you take a whale you give back the face to the sea, and the whale grows a new parka. It can only do it twice. After that it becomes another animal." The word *different* is often used to mean what we might term "on another level," but their word *different* is probably the best one.

Annie also termed the whale *different*. She said, "It talks to other whales; it knows if you are a good person."

"Other whales will surround an injured whale and pull it away with them," said Ed Tukumavik.

"Whales are ticklish," said Jeanne. "They don't like to see pregnant women down on the ice."

When I was visiting Louis's old grandfather Aklak, his nephew was preparing for a trip. "Is he going hunting?" I asked.

"I don't know," said the grandfather. "The animal will hear if you talk like that. If you say, 'I am going to kill a whale,' it will hear and something bad will happen. If you say, 'I am going down on the ice, and need some food to feed those poor people,' the animal will come to be caught."

16: Rich Parkas and Festival Food

1. In the anthropological research field, the experience of having natives question the anthropologists, turning the tables on them, stating their dislike of and opposition to the discipline, as Micky Hoffman also did at a later date, is becoming nearly universal. Who would want to be researched by an anthropologist? My reaction to this dilemma (and the reaction of many anthropologists today) is to patiently seek further understanding and

develop an attitude of respect. I appreciate the field people's view. They are all the time conscious, they are real people. In my view, our business now is to serve them, to act as a link for them, and if possible to serve the planet with knowledge generally, if knowledge on a broader scale will help.

2. This curing technique closely resembled the methods of extraction of many American Indian groups and other societies and, in certain ways, the African extraction of a wandering and afflicting tooth performed with cupping horns, like the one I witnessed in 1985 (E. Turner 1992).

17: The Whaling Festival

1. One of Victor Turner's tools of analysis of symbol and ritual (1967, 50, 52) was to find the positional level of meaning. That is, when in doubt as to the meaning of a symbol, one resort is to search the traditions for the positioning of that symbol in other aspects of the culture. Something of the meaning of an unknown symbol can then become clear.

2. By 1992 Michael's peroration had changed to: "In the old days the whale was our God. Now we are blending this idea with Christianity. But we must never forget our tradition. We must always continue whaling. . . . The whale was our God." Iñupiat traditions pointed to the whale as the being with the initiative, the one that caused the development of spirit awareness among human beings. The whale was also considered the mentor of morals and a being with self-determination that gave itself voluntarily for the benefit of humanity. The animals were greater than human beings (see Walens 1987). In mission times, assimilated Iñupiat who were following White teaching tended to erect "God" as the ruler of the whale and of all things. Now in contrast to the prayer of thanks in 1988, Michael was talking in 1992 about "blending," because his Iñupiat awareness had grown and was in the ascendancy. Jim Agnasagga drew my attention to this change in Michael, and Jim gained hope from the fact.

In both systems, Iñupiat and Christian, the hunt's success was not attributed to the virtues of human beings but to that of some spiritual being.

3. James Provenzano comments on the importance of the views of ethnic minorities in his article "Two Views of Ethnicity":

> The structural functionalist position of many social scientists puts them at odds with advocates seeking to alter the life situation of ethnic minority groups in America. . . . As ethnic groups combine to concern themselves with the development of ethnic consciousness as an adjunct to organization it becomes ever more necessary that social scientists make every effort to comprehend and incorporate the use of ideology by particular groups into the analytic tools devised to deal with these observed phenomena. (1976, 386)

He asserts that "social scientists whether Durkheimian, Marxists, or some other stripe, are being ignored by ethnic minorities not because we are racists or bigots, but because we are irrelevant to their problems" (1976, 400).

18: The Shaman's Four-Day Syndrome

1. All of Alaska's time is regulated in one time zone, although the state extends over three. This has been fixed to suit government and other agencies. Their reason is that because much of the north is sparsely populated, separate time zones are inappropriate and inefficient.

2. By 1991 Claire had taken her degree, mostly with A grades. She received an A for anthropology and also for Shakespeare, which she learned to love. She used to quote from *The Tempest*, and used a phrase referring to the afflictions of hell, appropriate for a shaman suffering strange episodes.

3. I am at a loss to say what kind of expert would be qualified to explain these cases. A psychologist? A psychic researcher? A neurobiologist? A scholar of religion? My own understanding is that there tends to exist a certain natural periodicity about the advent of a spirit, just as there exists a particular periodicity in pregnancy, nine months, nearly exactly; also, of course, there is a periodicity in our circadian physical processes. Biological periodicity in itself needs further study. Thomas Buckley (1988, 190) writes that menstruating women among the Yurok are said to "gain spiritual accomplishment" at the time of menstruation—often a four-day period. The question remains unanswered.

4. Eliade (1964, esp. 43–45) and others have described the shaman's dismemberment, "sparagmos," the breaking up of the person in the course of his or her shaman journey and subsequently becoming reassembled along with new powers.

5. Little Ezra did turn up in the village after a year or two and was in nursery school by 1993.

Conclusion

1. Compare what Yang (1994, 287–311) terms "rhizomatic networks," unofficial, non-kin networks of interpersonal help in China.

Bibliography

Abu-Lughod, Lila
1993   *Writing Women's Worlds.* Berkeley: University of California
        Press.
Babcock, Barbara
1974   "The Novel and the Carnival World." *Modern Languages Notes*
        89:911–37.
Bakhtin, Mikhail
1965   *Rabelais and His World.* Cambridge: MIT Press.
1981   *The Dialogic Imagination.* Austin: University of Texas Press.
Berger, Thomas
1985   *Village Journey: The Report of the Alaska Native Land Review
        Commission.* New York: Hill and Wang.
Berning, Karin
1986   "The Religious Aspect of the Kivggersuat or Messenger Feast."
        N.p.
Blackman, Margaret
1989   *Sadie Brower Neakok: An Iñupiaq Woman.* Seattle: University
        of Washington Press.
Bowen, Eleanor Smith
1954   *Return to Laughter.* New York: Harper.
Brady, Ivan
1991   *Anthropological Poetics.* Savage, Md.: Rowman and Littlefield.
Briggs, Jean L.
1970   *Never in Anger: Portrait of an Eskimo Family.* Cambridge: Har-
        vard University Press.
Brown, Karen McCarthy
1991   *Mama Lola: A Voudou Priestess in Brooklyn.* Berkeley: Univer-
        sity of California Press.
Buckley, Thomas
1988   "Menstruation and the Power of Yurok Women." In *Blood
        Magic: The Anthropology of Menstruation,* eds. Thomas Buckley
        and Alma Gottlieb, 187–209. Berkeley: University of Califor-
        nia Press.

Burch, Ernest S.
1971   "The Nonempirical Environment of the Arctic Alaskan Eski-
        mos." *Southwestern Journal of Anthropology* 27(2):148–65.
1975   *Eskimo Kinsmen.* St. Paul: West.
Chance, Norman
1966   *The Eskimos of Northern Alaska.* New York: Holt, Reinhart, and
        Winston.
Clifford, James
1983   "On Ethnographic Authority." *Representations* 1(2):118–46.
Desjarlais, Robert
1992   *Body and Emotion.* Philadelphia: University of Pennsylvania Press.
Devisch, René
1993   *Weaving the Threads of Life: The Khila Gyn-Eco-Logical Healing
        Cult among the Yaka.* Chicago: University of Chicago Press.
Eliade, Mircea
1964   *Shamanism: Archaic Techniques of Ecstasy.* Princeton, N.J.:
        Bollingen.
Evans-Pritchard, E. E.
1937   *Witchcraft, Oracles, and Magic among the Azande.* Oxford:
        Clarendon.
Fabian, Johannes
1983   *Time and the Other.* New York: Columbia University Press.
Favret-Saada, Jeanne
1980   *Deadly Words: Witchcraft in the Bocage.* Cambridge: Cambridge
        University Press.
Fienup-Riordan, Ann
1983   *The Nelson Island Eskimo.* Anchorage: Alaska Pacific University
        Press.
1990   *Eskimo Essays.* New Brunswick: Rutgers University Press.
1994   *Boundaries and Passages: Rule and Ritual in Yup'ik Eskimo
        Oral Tradition.* Norman: University of Oklahoma Press.
Fitzhugh, William W., and Aron Crowell
1988   *Crossroads of Continents: Cultures of Siberia and Alaska.* Wash-
        ington, DC: Smithsonian Institution Press.
Foulks, Edward F.
1972   *The Arctic Hysterias of the Alaskan Eskimo.* Washington: Ameri-
        can Anthropological Association.
Gleick, James
1987   *Chaos: Making a New Science.* New York: Viking.
Goulet, Jean-Guy
1994   "Ways of Knowing: Towards a Narrative Ethnography of Expe-
        riences among the Dene Tha." *Journal of Anthropological Re-
        search* 50(2):113–39.
Graves, Robert, and Raphael Patai
1966   *Hebrew Myths: The Book of Genesis.* New York: McGraw-Hill.
Grindal, Bruce
1983   "Into the Heart of Sisala Experience: Witnessing Death Divina-

tion." *Journal of Anthropological Research* 39(1):60–80.

Guédon, Francoise-Marie
1994   "Dene Ways and the Ethnographer's Culture." In *Being Changed by Cross-Cultural Encounters: The Anthropology of Extraordinary Experience,* eds. David Young and Jean-Guy Goulet, 39–70. Peterborough, Ontario: Broadview.

Hultkrantz, Åke
1992   *Shamanic Healing and Ritual Drama.* New York: Crossroads.

Iñupiat Community of the Arctic Slope
1979   *The Iñupiat View.* Anchorage: U.S. Department of the Interior, National Petroleum Reserve in Alaska, 105 (c). Final Studies, vol. l(b).

Jackson, Michael
1989   *Paths toward a Clearing: Radical Empiricism and Ethnographic Inquiry.* Bloomington: Indiana University Press.

James, William
1976   *Essays in Radical Empiricism.* Cambridge: Harvard University Press.

Juul, Sandra
1979   "Portrait of an Eskimo Tribal Doctor." *Alaska Medicine* 21(6):66–71.

King, Stanley Hall
1962   *Perceptions of Illness and Medical Practice.* New York: Russell Sage Foundation.

Kingsley, Charles
1928 [1863]   *The Water Babies.* Reprint, London: Macmillan.

Kondo, Dorinne
1990   *Crafting Selves.* Chicago: University of Chicago Press.

Laderman, Carol
1991   *Taming the Winds of Desire.* Berkeley: University of California Press.

Lantis, Margaret
1947   *Alaskan Eskimo Ceremonialism.* Seattle: University of Washington Press.

Laughlin, Charles
1994   "Apodicticity: The Problem of Absolute Certainty in Transpersonal Ethnography." *Anthropology and Humanism* 19(2):115–29.

Lavie, Smadar
1990   *The Poetics of Military Occupation.* Berkeley: University of California Press.

Lévi-Strauss, Claude
1963   *Structuralism.* New York: Basic Books.

Lévy-Bruhl, Lucien
1985 [1910]   *How Natives Think.* Reprint, Princeton: Princeton University Press.

Lucier, Charles, James Vanstone, and Della Keats
1971   "Medical Practices and Human Anatomical Knowledge among the Noatak Eskimos." *Ethnology* 10(3):251–64.

MacClean, Edna Ahgeak
1980   *Iñupiallu Tanngillu Uqalungisa Ilangich: Abridged Iñupiaq and English Dictionary.* Fairbanks: University of Alaska.

Marton, Yves
1994   "The Experiential Approach to Anthropology." In *Being Changed by Cross-Cultural Encounters: The Anthropology of Extraordinary Experience,* eds. David Young and Jean-Guy Goulet, 273–97. Peterborough, Ontario: Broadview.

Mauss, Marcel
1954   *The Gift: Forms and Functions of Exchange in Archaic Societies.* Trans. Ian Cunnison. London: Cohen and West.

McCall, John
1993   "Making Peace with Agwu." *Anthropology and Humanism* 18(2):56–66.

Merkur, Daniel
1985   *Becoming Half-Hidden: Shamanism and Initiation among the Inuit.* Stockholm: Almqvist and Wiksell.

Moody, Raymond A.
1976   *Life after Life: The Investigation of a Phenomenon—Survival of Bodily Death.* New York: Bantam.

Myerhoff, Barbara
1978   "Return to Wirikuta: Ritual Reversal and Symbolic Continuity on the Peyote Hunt of the Huichol Indians." In *The Reversible World: Symbolic Inversion in Art and Society,* ed. Barbara Myerhoff, 225–39. Ithaca, N.Y.: Cornell University Press.

Narayan, Kirin
1989   *Storytellers, Saints, and Scoundrels: Folk Narrative in Hindu Religious Teaching.* Philadelphia: University of Pennsylvania Press.

Nelson, Richard
1983   *Make Prayers to Raven.* Chicago: University of Chicago Press.

Obeyesekere, Gananath
N.D.   *Imagining Karma: Ethical Consummation in Amerindian, Buddhist, and Greek Rebirth.* Forthcoming.

Oquilluk, William
1981   *People of Kauwerak.* Anchorage: Alaska Pacific University Press.

Peters, Larry
1981   *Ecstacy and Healing in Nepal: An Ethnopsychiatric Study of Tamang Shamanism.* Malibu Calif.: Undena Publications.

Provenzano, James
1976   "Two Views of Ethnicity." In *Ethnicity in the Americas,* ed. Frances Henry, 305–404. The Hague: Mouton.

Rassmusen, Knut
1952 [1923–1924]   *The Alaskan Eskimos.* Reprint, Copenhagen: Gyldendal.

Ray, Dorothy Jean, and Alfred A. Blaker
1967   *Eskimo Masks: Art and Ceremony.* Seattle: University of Washington Press.

Rose, Dan
1991   "Reversal." In *Anthropological Poetics,* ed. Ivan Brady, 283–301. Savage, Md.: Rowman and Littlefield.

Saladin-d'Anglure, Bernard
1990   "Frère-lune (Taqqiq), soeur-soleil (Siqiniq) et l'intelligence du monde (Sila): Cosmologie inuit, cosmographie arctique et espace-temps chamanique" (Brother moon, sister sun, and the intelligence of the world: From arctic cosmography to Inuit cosmology). *Études/Inuit/Studies* 14(1–2):75–140.

Salamone, Frank
1995   "The Bori and I: Reflections of a Mature Anthropologist." *Anthropology and Humanism* 20(1):15–19.

Sharp, H. Stephen
1987   "Giant Fish, Giant Otters, and Dinosaurs: 'Apparently Irrational' Beliefs in a Chipewyan Community." *American Ethnologist* 14(2):226–35.

1994   "Inverted Sacrifice." In *Circumpolar Religion and Ecology,* eds. Takashi Irimoto and Takako Yamada, 253–72. Tokyo: University of Tokyo Press.

Søby, Regitze Margrethe
1990   "The Kalaaq Story: Same Name—Same Destiny." Paper Presented at the Seventh Inuit Studies Conference, Aug. 19–23, Fairbanks.

Spencer, R. F.
1959   *The North Alaska Eskimo: A Study in Ecology and Society.* Bureau of American Ethnology Bulletin 171. Washington, D.C.

Stoller, Paul
1989   *The Taste of Ethnographic Things.* Philadelphia: University of Pennsylvania Press.

Taussig, Michael
1987   *Shamanism, Colonialism, and the Wild Man: A Study in Terror and Healing.* Chicago: University of Chicago Press.

Tedlock, Dennis
1990   *Days from a Dream Almanac.* Urbana: University of Illinois Press.

Trawick, Margaret
1990   *Notes on Love in a Tamil Family.* Berkeley: University of California Press.

Turner, Edith
1986   "Philip Kabwita, Ghost Doctor: The Ndembu in 1985." *Drama Review* 30(4):4–45.

1992   *Experiencing Ritual: A New Interpretation of African Healing* (with William Blodgett, Singleton Kahona, and Fideli Benwa). Philadelphia: University of Pennsylvania Press.

Turner, Victor
1967   *The Forest of Symbols.* Ithaca, N.Y.: Cornell University Press.
1969   *The Ritual Process: Structure and Anti-Structure.* Chicago: Aldine.
1974   *Dramas, Fields, and Metaphors.* Ithaca, N.Y.: Cornell University Press.
1975   *Revelation and Divination.* Ithaca, N.Y.: Cornell University Press.
1986   "Dewey, Dilthey, and Drama: An Essay in the Anthropology of Experience." In *The Anthropology of Experience,* eds. Victor Turner and Edward Bruner, 33–44. Urbana: University of Illinois Press.

Turner, Victor, and Edward Bruner, eds.
1986   *The Anthropology of Experience.* Urbana: University of Illinois Press.

Wafer, James
1991   *A Taste of Blood: Spirit Possession in Brazilian Candomblé.* Philadelphia: University of Pennsylvania Press.

Wagner, Roy
1986   *Symbols that Stand for Themselves.* Chicago: University of Chicago Press.

Walens, Stanley
1981   *Feasting with Cannibals: An Essay on Kwakiutl Cosmology.* Princeton: Princeton University Press.
1987   "Animals." In *Encyclopedia of Religion,* eds. Mircea Eliade et al. vol. 1, 291–96. New York: Macmillan.

Winkelman, Michael
1992   *Shamans, Priests, and Witches: A Cross-Cultural Study of Magico-Religious Practitioners.* Tempe: Arizona State University Press.

Wooley, Chris, and Rex Okakak
1989   "Kivgiq: A Celebration of Who We Are." Paper presented at the 16th Annual Meeting of the Alaska Anthropological Association, March 3–4, Anchorage.

Yang, Mayfair Mei-hui
1994   *Gifts, Favors, and Banquets: The Art of Social Relationships in China.* Ithaca, N.Y.: Cornell University Press.

Young, David
1994   "Visitors in the Night: A Creative Energy Model of Spontaneous Visions." In *Being Changed by Cross-Cultural Encounters: The Anthropology of Extraordinary Experience,* eds. David Young and Jean-Guy Goulet, 166–94. Peterborough, Ontario: Broadview.

Young, David, and Jean-Guy Goulet, eds.
1994   *Being Changed by Cross-Cultural Encounters: The Anthropology of Extraordinary Experience.* Peterborough, Ontario: Broadview.

Index